The Johns Hopkins White Papers

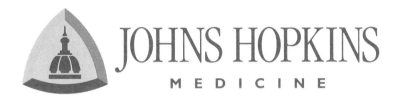

JOHNS HOPKINS
M E D I C I N E

Depression and Anxiety

Your personal guide to prevention, diagnosis and treatment

Karen L. Swartz, M.D.

2012

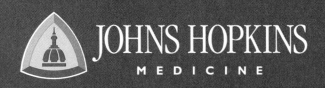

JOHNS HOPKINS
M E D I C I N E

The Johns Hopkins White Papers are a series of disease-specific publications designed for health care consumers with chronic conditions who desire accurate, comprehensive and easy-to-understand information to enable them to better manage their disorder. Each White Paper is prepared in consultation with one or more specialists from Johns Hopkins Medicine. A new, updated edition of each White Paper is released each January and sold throughout the year.

The White Papers are produced in partnership with Remedy Health Media, LLC. For information on our complete line of Johns Hopkins health publications—our White Papers and Digital Special Reports, our Prostate and Memory Bulletins, and our monthly Health After 50 newsletter—please visit our website: **www.JohnsHopkinsHealthAlerts.com.**

Basic price: $39.95

ISBN 978-1-935584-51-3

Printed in the United States of America

The information contained in this White Paper is not intended as a substitute for the advice of a physician. Readers who suspect they may have specific medical problems should consult a physician about any suggestions made.

The Johns Hopkins White Papers

Esther Benenson
Editor in Chief, Digital & Print
Johns Hopkins Publications

Joanne Gallo
Executive Editor

Michael Brady
Christina Frank
Devon Schuyler
Staff Writers

Kimberly Flynn
Contributing Writer

Kimberly Flynn
Editorial Research

Tim Jeffs
Creative Director

Dragonfly Media Group
Medical Illustrations

Joyce Ippolito
Copy Editor

Remedy Health Media, LLC

Traver Hutchins
Chairman

Michael Cunnion
Chief Executive Officer

David Lee
Executive Vice President, Publishing

Patrick Aysseh
Executive Vice President, Digital

Lisa Cohen
Chief Financial Officer

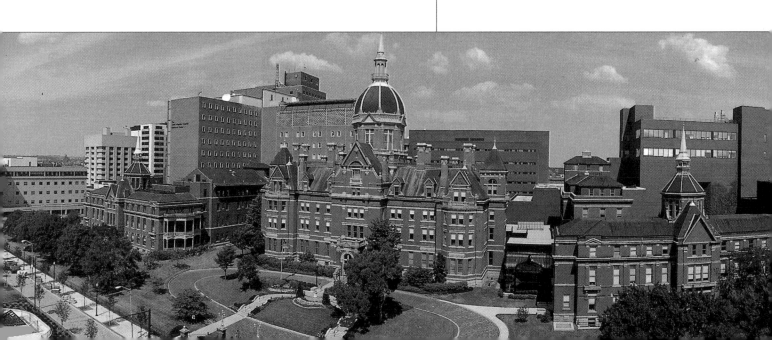

Table of Contents

Introducing Your
Depression and Anxiety Expert

The Johns Hopkins Hospital is No. 1 in the United States for psychiatry, according to U.S. News & World Report's Best Hospitals rankings for 2011-12. Your Johns Hopkins expert for the Depression and Anxiety White Paper is Dr. Karen L. Swartz.

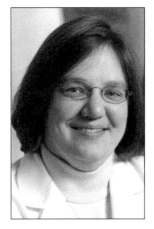

Karen L. Swartz, M.D., is the Director of Clinical and Educational Programs at the Johns Hopkins Mood Disorders Center and is an Associate Professor in the Department of Psychiatry and Behavioral Sciences at the Johns Hopkins School of Medicine. She is also Codirector of the Women's Mood Disorders Center and is a recognized expert on the subject of premenstrual dysphoric disorder, mood disorders during pregnancy, postpartum depression and psychosis, and menopause-related depression. She is the Founder and Director of the Adolescent Depression Awareness Program (ADAP), a school-based depression education program for students, faculty and parents. Dr. Swartz has also written articles for such journals as *Archives of General Psychiatry, Current Opinion in Psychiatry,* the *International Review of Psychiatry* and the *Journal of the American Academy of Child and Adolescent Psychiatry.*

Depression and Anxiety

Elation, sadness, anxiety, grief—we all feel these emotions at various times in our lives. Sadness may be caused by a setback or a loss, while anxiety may be triggered by a threat or a challenge. It is perfectly natural for our emotions to wax and wane with the ups and downs of our lives. The difficulty comes when these feelings do not go away—or when they seemingly occur out of the blue without explanation—and begin to interfere with our daily functioning. When that's the case, a mood disorder, such as depression or bipolar disorder, or an anxiety disorder may be present.

In any given year, about one in four Americans develops at least one mental health disorder. Depression and other mental health disorders were responsible for 156 million visits to doctors, clinics, and hospital outpatient departments in 2005. Fortunately, effective treatments are available. Proper diagnosis and treatment of mood disorders lead to a remission of symptoms in about 80 percent of cases. This White Paper provides detailed information on the causes, symptoms, diagnoses and treatments of depression, bipolar disorder and anxiety disorders.

MOOD DISORDERS

Depression and bipolar disorder are commonly referred to as mood (affective) disorders. Major hallmarks of depression include a persistent low or sad mood, decreased or absent interest in almost all activities, loss of self-confidence and a feeling of worthlessness. Most people with bipolar disorder, formerly known as manic-depressive illness, experience alternating episodes of depression and mania. Mania, which can be thought of as the opposite of depression, is characterized by an elated or elevated mood, increased activity, an overblown self-image and an exaggerated sense of self-confidence. Usually, both depression and bipolar disorder are episodic—that is, bouts of illness are separated by symptom-free periods characterized by feelings of relative well-being.

Causes of Mood Disorders

The exact causes of depression and bipolar disorder are not well understood, but some combination of genetic predisposition and psychological and medical factors appears to play a role in these disorders.

Changes in the Brain

The brain is composed of distinct regions, each made up of networks of nerve cells (neurons) that transmit messages throughout the nervous system. Individual neurons are separated by small gaps at each end called synaptic clefts. Chemicals called neurotransmitters bridge the synaptic clefts and pass messages from one neuron to the next. Imbalances in three particular neurotransmitters—serotonin, norepinephrine and dopamine—appear to contribute to depression and bipolar disorder, although less is known about changes in the brain that occur during the manic phase of bipolar disorder.

One specific brain region thought to be involved in depression is the limbic system, which affects our emotional behavior. An area within this system, the hypothalamus, regulates the pituitary gland, which in turn regulates key hormones and may be involved in the hormonal imbalances sometimes associated with depression (see the illustration on page 3).

Genetic Factors

Depression is often a family affair. Scientists, for example, have identified a gene that may be linked to bipolar disorder. In addition, they have found a common genetic mutation associated with clinical depression after a traumatic event.

Research also shows that when one identical twin has a mood disorder, there is about a 50 percent chance that the other twin, who shares the same genes, will develop the illness at some point in life. One study found that if one twin developed depression, the other twin also suffered from depression in 46 percent of identical twins, compared with 20 percent of fraternal twins (who share half of their genes, like any full siblings).

Studies have also found that adopted children whose biological parents had a mood disorder had a three times greater incidence of depressive illness than the biological children of the same adoptive parents. Finally, children whose parents and grandparents experienced moderate to severe depression are at much greater risk for developing psychiatric problems than those whose relatives were

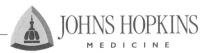

Anatomy of the Brain

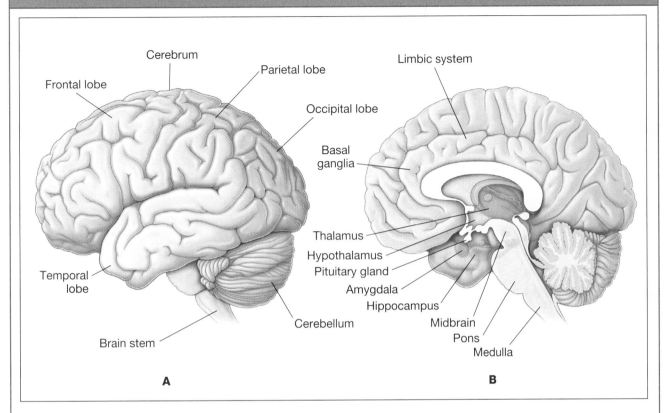

A

B

The brain is composed of several distinct regions, and each has certain specialized functions (A). Brain function is extremely complex, and new information about the parts of the brain and how they work is continually being discovered. This illustration represents a very simplified description of brain function.

The brainstem (formed by the medulla, pons, and midbrain) links the spinal cord to the higher parts of the brain, acting as a conduit for the nerves going to and coming from the body. It is also involved in the control of basic functions, such as breathing and blood pressure. The cerebellum controls muscle coordination and balance and plays a role in memory. The cerebrum—the largest portion of the brain—is divided into two distinct hemispheres, each comprised of a frontal, parietal, occipital and temporal lobe. It is the center of consciousness, intellect, memory and language, among other functions. The diencephalon, which lies inside the cerebrum, consists of the thalamus and the hypothalamus. The diencephalon and the midbrain also play a part in consciousness, memory and intellect.

Scientists believe that disorders like depression or anxiety may result from chemical imbalances that affect the limbic system, the basal ganglia and the circuits that are part of the basal ganglia (B). The limbic system is a group of structures, including the frontal lobe cerebral cortex (the cortex is the outer layer of the cerebrum), temporal lobe, thalamus, hypothalamus, amygdala, hippocampus and the network of nerves that connects them to each other. The thalamus acts as a relay station for passing all sensory impulses except smell into the cerebrum. The hypothalamus controls body temperature, appetite, water balance, sexual behavior and other body functions, and plays a central part in certain emotions as well. It also regulates the pituitary gland, and may be involved with the hormonal imbalance that is sometimes associated with depression. The amygdala controls fear, rage and aggression, and is connected to the parts of the brainstem that regulate heart rate, perspiration and breathing. It may play an important role in anxiety disorders, which arise because of an inability to control fear. The hippocampus acts as a memory center, matching new information with that already stored in the brain. The basal ganglia are a group of complex, interconnected structures that are linked by circuits to the cortex and the thalamus. ■

not affected, according to a three-generation study.

Genetics also plays a role in treatment, influencing an individual's response to a particular drug, for example. There is evidence that people may do better if prescribed the same antidepressant medication that has been effective for a depressed first-degree relative (a parent, sibling or child).

Because researchers are not sure exactly which genes are linked to depression or bipolar disorder, specific genetic tests will not be available for years to come. But as with heart disease and cancer, it is important to know if you have a family history of depression or bipolar disorder.

Although genetic factors may make a person more susceptible to mood disorders, a trigger—such as a serious medical condition or psychological stress—is often what causes a mood disorder to emerge at a specific time.

Drugs and Alcohol

Overconsumption of alcohol and certain illegal drugs can contribute to depression and make it worse, as can withdrawal from alcohol, cocaine or amphetamines. Drugs can cause other mental changes as well. For example, amphetamines, cocaine and phencyclidine (PCP) can all induce mania in people with bipolar disorder.

Medical Conditions

Medical disorders can make people prone to depression. For example, people who have dementia-causing brain disorders, such as Alzheimer's disease or Huntington's disease, are more susceptible to depression. In addition, stroke is known to trigger depression, affecting about 25 percent of those who have had a stroke in the left frontal area of the brain.

Hormonal disorders, such as an underactive thyroid (hypothyroidism) and Cushing's disease (in which the adrenal gland produces too much of the stress hormone cortisol, affecting blood pressure and metabolism) also can lead to depression. A recent study suggests that low testosterone levels may be responsible for an increase in depression in men after age 65.

Vitamin deficiencies, such as insufficient levels of folic acid, vitamin B_6 or vitamin B_{12}, also have been linked to depression. In one study of 700 women, those with a vitamin B_{12} deficiency were twice as likely to be severely depressed as those without this deficiency.

Two recent studies suggest that obese adults may be more likely to develop a mental health disorder, and those with metabolic

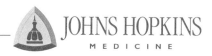

syndrome (a combination of excess weight, high cholesterol, high blood glucose levels and high blood pressure) are also at increased risk.

Medication

Prescription drugs also can cause mood disorders. Medications such as corticosteroids, levodopa (Parcopa and other drugs used to treat Parkinson's disease) and methylphenidate (Ritalin and others commonly used for treating attention deficit disorder) can trigger mania in bipolar disorder. Other drugs, including some used to treat high blood pressure and cancer, have been known to cause depression.

Brain Trauma

Neurological disorders or injury to the brain from trauma or tumors can cause behavioral changes, anxiety and/or mood disorders.

Symptoms and Diagnosis of Mood Disorders

Although many mood disorders are readily recognized, it can be difficult to distinguish milder forms of depression or anxiety from the emotional changes that are part of everyday life. Unlike most medical conditions, mood disorders cannot be detected by blood and other laboratory tests. Rather, a doctor must rely on a person's medical history to diagnose a mood disorder.

The American Psychiatric Association has established a classification system to help doctors make consistent diagnoses of major depression, bipolar disorder and various forms of anxiety. These criteria are defined in the *Diagnostic and Statistical Manual of Mental Disorders*, a reference guide used by psychiatrists, psychologists, and other mental health professionals. The manual is periodically revised to keep up with the latest research. The current edition is referred to as the *DSM-IV-TR*.

Major Depression

In any given year, 15 million American adults—approximately 5 to 8 percent of the population—suffers at least one episode of major depression, and only 60 percent of these individuals reportedly receive treatment. According to the *DSM-IV-TR*, a person is suffering from a major depressive episode if he or she experiences items

1 or 2 from the list of symptoms below, along with any four others, for more than two weeks:

1. Depressed mood with overwhelming feelings of sadness and grief
2. Apathy—loss of interest and pleasure in activities formerly enjoyed
3. Sleep problems—insomnia, early-morning waking or oversleeping nearly every day
4. Decreased energy or fatigue
5. Noticeable changes in appetite and weight (significant weight loss or gain)
6. Inability to concentrate or think, or indecisiveness
7. Physical symptoms of restlessness or being physically slowed down
8. Feelings of guilt, worthlessness, and helplessness
9. Recurrent thoughts of death or suicide, or a suicide attempt

The diagnosis is more certain when a person has a family history of depression, has had a previous episode of depression or bipolar disorder, has a general medical problem likely to trigger depression (such as a recent stroke or heart attack), or is taking a medication known to cause mood disorders.

Other symptoms of depression include disorganized thinking and delusions. In addition to these disturbances in mood and cognition (thinking), people with major depression may experience physical changes such as constipation or decreased sexual drive.

Episodes of major depression range from mild to severe. In mild episodes, symptoms barely meet the requirements for a diagnosis and the person is able to get through the day without much trouble. Severe episodes are characterized by several debilitating symptoms, including worsening mood that markedly interferes with daily life. People struggling with severe depression have difficulty with almost every activity—going to work, socializing and even getting up in the morning. In the most severe cases, depressed individuals may be unable to feed and dress themselves or maintain personal hygiene.

Major depression is believed to be twice as common in women as in men, although that statistic is now being questioned. In fact, depression symptoms may be different in men and women, as well as in older versus younger people. Men are more inclined to get angry and irritable, feel an increasing loss of control over their lives, take greater risks, become more aggressive and complain about problems at work rather than feeling sad, weepy, worthless or guilty, as women usually do.

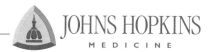

Dysthymia

Dysthymia is a chronic form of depression that is milder than major depression. It is characterized by the presence of depressed mood for most of the day, for more days than not, over a period of at least two years. It may be intermittent and interspersed with periods of feeling normal, but these periods of improvement last no more than two months.

Dysthymia is believed to be twice as common in women as in men. People who have dysthymia before age 21 tend to have a higher incidence of personality disorders. Because the onset of symptoms is insidious, dysthymia often goes unnoticed. And because of its chronic nature, the person may come to believe that he or she had always been that way. In addition to depressed mood, symptoms include two or more of the following:
- Poor appetite or overeating
- Insomnia or hypersomnia (excessive sleeping)
- Low energy or fatigue
- Low self-esteem
- Poor concentration or difficulty making decisions
- Feelings of hopelessness

It is far better to treat dysthymia than to think of it as a minor condition. Bypassing treatment places people at increased risk of subsequently developing major depression. In fact, about 10 percent of people with dysthymia have recurrent episodes of major depression, a condition known as double depression.

Biological causes

Some medical conditions, including neurological disorders (such as multiple sclerosis and stroke), hypothyroidism, fibromyalgia and chronic fatigue syndrome, are associated with dysthymia. Investigators believe that, in these cases, developing dysthymia is not a psychological reaction to being ill but rather is a biological effect of these disorders. There are many reasons for this connection. It may be that these medical conditions interfere with the action of neurotransmitters, that medications (such as corticosteroids or beta-blockers) taken for a medical illness may trigger the dysthymia, or that both dysthymia and the medical illness are related in some other way, reinforcing each other in a complicated manner.

Dysthymia can also follow severe psychological stress, such as losing a spouse or caring for a chronically ill loved one. Older people who have never had psychiatric disorders are particularly susceptible to developing dysthymia after significant life stresses.

Atypical Depression

Atypical depression, despite its name, is not unusual and occurs in 25 to 40 percent of depressed patients. However, it differs from typical depression in certain key respects. For example, sufferers do manage to find pleasure in certain activities at certain times, and, rather than having insomnia and loss of appetite, many people with atypical depression overeat and oversleep.

Other symptoms include:
- A general sadness that can be interrupted by enjoyment of pleasurable experiences or circumstances
- Strong feelings of rejection
- A sensation of heaviness, especially in the arms
- A strong preference to overeat carbohydrate-rich foods because ingestion of carbohydrates causes an increase in serotonin in the brain, which can boost mood

The disorder can be just as debilitating as the more traditional forms of major depression. People with atypical depression often have shorter—but more frequent— episodes of depression.

Seasonal Affective Disorder (SAD)

As the seasons change, so does the amount of sunlight each day. This in turn causes changes in people's internal biological clocks (also called circadian rhythm). This rhythm is a 24-hour cycle that affects our eating and sleeping patterns as well as biological activities such as brain wave activity, hormone production and cell regeneration. In some individuals, less daily sunlight and changes in circadian rhythm can induce depression, which usually peaks in January and February, when there is the least sunlight. Researchers believe that the lack of sunlight during these times may alter brain levels of certain mood-controlling substances. For example, the hormone melatonin may decrease.

People with SAD often eat and sleep excessively, crave sugary or starchy foods and have a full remission in the spring and summer, when more daily sunlight is available.

Grief Versus Depression

Sometimes we experience huge changes in our lives. These events can cause intense emotional anguish, and grieving during such life changes is a normal and healthy—if painful—process. Grief can be the result of a major life change, such as:
- The death of a loved one (a person or pet)
- A move to a new and unfamiliar community

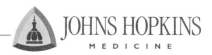

- An opportunity or life goal that becomes closed to us
- A loved one contracting a life-threatening illness

Occasionally, however, this anguish triggers a major depressive episode, although few people in mourning experience true clinical depression.

Even a serious illness can increase the risk of stress and, potentially, depression in a partner: A recent study of 518,000 couples over age 65 found that when one spouse was hospitalized for a serious illness, the other spouse had a greater risk of dying within the next year. The probable reasons were increased stress and withdrawal of social, emotional, economic and other support.

Grieving often produces a wide range of feelings. The psychological process itself is a way for the mind to adjust, over time, to the acute sorrow of a loss. Grieving also allows us to accept the finality of the loss, to experience a full range of feelings as a result of the loss, and to adjust to our changed lives. The end of grieving does not entail forgetting; rather, it usually comes with the acceptance of our loss.

A good sign that mourning is successful is a gradual shift from sad thoughts and feelings to thoughts of positive and realistic plans for the future. As this shift occurs over time and the mourner begins to enjoy life more than feeling weighed down by it, the process of grieving moves forward.

Although grief and depression may both entail feeling sad, they are different. The sadness of grief usually comes in "waves," with varying degrees of intensity and bouts of crying, and intense feelings of sadness, guilt, anger, irritability or loneliness. An individual experiencing grief, however, can enjoy some of life's activities. Grief is generally temporary and resolves without specific treatment.

Depression is a more persistent and unremitting sadness and is notable for a consistent inability to enjoy pleasurable life activities. Muted or "deadened" feelings are often a sign of depression. If such symptoms persist following a life change that produces grief, mourning may have been unsuccessful and the help of a physician or other health professional is warranted. Check for the following symptoms, especially over a prolonged period or if they arise months or even years after the loss:

- Physical symptoms that mimic the illness or injury of the person who died
- Overuse of alcohol, illegal drugs or prescription drugs
- Persistent depression (see page 5 for symptoms)
- Chronic sleep disturbances

- Thoughts of or attempts at suicide (see a health professional immediately)
- Inability to carry out normal daily routines

It is important to seek medical help for physical symptoms that arise during mourning and to address any medical or psychiatric conditions that existed before the death occurred. Some evidence suggests that acute mourning may suppress the immune system and make people more susceptible to illness.

Depression in Older Adults

Depression and aging do not necessarily go hand in hand. A survey of Californians ages 50 to 95 found that factors such as chronic illness, physical disabilities and social isolation—which often coincide with increasing age—were stronger predictors of depression than age itself. That said, the incidence of depression is clearly higher in older adults. An estimated 6.5 million of the nation's 35 million people age 65 and older suffer from major depression. Unfortunately, the disease is often undiagnosed, misdiagnosed or left untreated in the elderly and can increase the risk of early death and repeated hospitalization. There is also reason to believe that late-life depression can be more serious than depression in younger people.

One reason depression may go undiagnosed is because of life circumstances that are common as we age, such as the loss of a spouse, family members or friends (due to death or geographic relocation); retirement, which may be accompanied by a loss of status and self-identity; financial concerns; fears of death or loss of independence; social isolation; and medical problems. Any of these factors may trigger symptoms of depression that are mistakenly attributed to life stresses and are not recognized as a true depressive illness.

Many older people who live alone do not have adequate support networks. Some don't know where to find help or are overwhelmed by the many resources providing medical care, social services and financial assistance. Older adults tend to be embarrassed or reluctant to seek professional help for emotional problems, partly because the stigma of psychiatric illness is especially strong among people in this age group, and/or because they remember the days when treatments were less effective. In addition, friends and family often fail to perceive signs of distress. Older depressed people are more likely to tell their primary care physician about physical complaints than about subjective feelings of depressed mood. For example, they may report loss of appetite, insomnia or lack of energy but not a loss of interest or enjoyment in daily activities. Unfortunately, doctors and patients alike often consider these symptoms a normal part of aging.

Because older people often have other medical illnesses and take more prescription drugs, it can take some medical sleuthing to accurately pin down a diagnosis of depression. Depression might be the primary disorder, a reaction to a prescription drug or the result of an underlying condition such as cancer or a stroke. It also might be a psychological reaction to a diagnosis of a serious illness or debilitating chronic pain or impairment. Finally, it could be a direct or indirect biological effect of an illness on the brain.

The possibility of dementia adds further difficulties. Symptoms of major depression can mimic those of a dementia-causing condition such as Alzheimer's disease (disorientation, distractibility and memory loss, for example). Doctors need to evaluate an individual's mental status, medical history and current physical health status carefully to find the primary cause of the psychological symptoms.

Effects of Depression on Physical Health

Depression clearly has a harmful effect on physical health, although the biological reasons for the link between body and mind are unclear. It may be that depression affects health because people develop a fatalistic attitude and stop taking care of themselves. Whatever the reasons, over the past 20 years it has become evident that a depressed mood after a heart attack is much more than an "understandable emotional reaction" to a stressful, life-changing event—it is profoundly dangerous, raising a person's chances of having a second, fatal heart attack. In fact, one recent study found that people with depression who suffer a heart attack are at increased risk for complications while still in the hospital.

More recently, researchers have studied the flip side of the equation—the question of whether someone who is depressed is at increased risk for developing coronary heart disease (CHD) down the line. Indeed, prospective studies show that people who had no CHD but were depressed when the studies began were more likely to develop or die of heart disease. A Norwegian study found that people with significant depression had a higher risk of dying of most major causes of death, even after adjusting for age, medical conditions and physical complaints.

Depression also aggravates chronic illnesses such as diabetes, arthritis, back problems and asthma, leading to more work absences, disability and doctor visits (see "Depression and Diabetes" on pages 14-15).

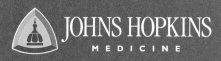

LATEST RESEARCH

Clues Help Predict Depression in Older People

Among older people with major depression, several factors may predict whether the depression will still be a problem six months later.

In a recent study, researchers from Boston analyzed data from 792 people ages 65 and older who had major depression. The participants took part in a study that compared different approaches for providing mental health services and measured how many people had remission from their major depression at six months.

Twenty-nine percent of participants experienced remission from their depression, and 71 percent did not. Factors that were associated with a higher chance of not responding included also having anxiety (linked to a 60 percent higher risk of non-remission), being female (49 percent higher risk), having medical problems (15 percent higher risk) and having more severe depression symptoms at the beginning (4 percent higher risk).

These findings support the idea that older people with depression along with other psychiatric or physical problems should be closely monitored.

INTERNATIONAL JOURNAL OF GERIATRIC PSYCHIATRY
Volume 26, page 48
January 2011

Bipolar Disorder

Bipolar disorder strikes men and women equally and affects about 3 percent of American adults at some point in their lives. A person with bipolar disorder typically has alternating periods of major depression and mania. In rare cases, mania can occur on its own.

Manic episodes are characterized by distinct periods of abnormally and persistently elevated or irritable mood. These episodes, with their restless energy and volatile mood swings, are severe enough to cause trouble at work, home or both. Episodes of milder manic symptoms are termed hypomania. Men with bipolar disorder tend to have more manic episodes; women are more likely to experience depressive episodes. The time between cycles can vary greatly (see "Natural History and Prognosis of Mood Disorders" on page 16).

Bipolar disorder can begin with an episode of either depression or mania, but about two-thirds of all cases start with a manic episode, and mania tends to predominate. A manic episode is accompanied by at least three of the following seven symptoms:

- Feelings of grandiosity or inflated self-esteem
- Diminished need for sleep
- Being extremely talkative
- The sense that thoughts and ideas are racing
- Being easily distracted
- Increased productivity and/or activity at work, at school or in social situations
- Excessive involvement in high-risk activities that are likely to have serious consequences

Because manic episodes can cause impaired judgment, people must be protected from engaging in self-destructive actions, such as making unwise investments, going on large spending or gambling sprees, driving recklessly or impulsively starting intense and unwise romantic or sexual relationships.

Certain medications and health conditions can cause significant mood swings that mimic the symptoms of bipolar disorder. These include corticosteroids, antidepressant or anti-anxiety drugs, drugs for Parkinson's disease such as tolcapone (Tasmar), abuse of alcohol or other drugs, an underactive or overactive thyroid gland, a neurological or adrenal disorder, vitamin B_{12} deficiency and other mental health conditions, such as schizophrenia. These potential causes of mood swings should be taken into account when a person is suspected of having bipolar disorder or is not responding to treatment.

Suicide

Suicide—the eighth leading cause of death in the United States—is a major complication of depression. About 7 percent of men and 1 percent of women diagnosed with depression die by suicide. Approximately two-thirds of all people who die by suicide are depressed. Ninety percent of those who die by suicide have a diagnosable psychiatric disorder.

In the United States, suicide risk is highest in older white and American Indian/Alaskan males and in those who live alone, have made prior suicide attempts, refuse psychiatric evaluation or abuse alcohol or other drugs. Although women attempt suicide three times more often than men, men are four times more likely to die by suicide. One study found that older people with a serious physical illness were six times more likely to die by suicide than those without an illness. In a U.K. study, interpersonal problems and bereavement, along with chronic physical illness (pain, breathlessness and functional limitation), were commonly associated with suicide in older people.

The risk of suicide is particularly high in people with untreated bipolar disorder. About 25 to 50 percent of those with the condition attempt suicide at least once. Moreover, suicide is a major concern among adolescents and young adults—it is the third leading cause of death among people ages 15 to 24.

Up to two-thirds of people who die by suicide visited their medical doctor in the prior month. This statistic suggests that they were aware that something was wrong but that neither they nor their doctor identified depression as the problem. Although it is impossible to predict accurately who will attempt suicide, there are warning signs that a severely depressed person may make an attempt. All too often, friends and relatives of people who die by suicide are unaware of these red flags until it is too late.

The most important steps to prevent suicide are to recognize the risk factors and warning signs and to facilitate appropriate treatment of the underlying psychiatric illness. New treatment guidelines call for people with major depression to have a careful and ongoing evaluation of their suicide risk. Typical warning signs are listed below. However, not all people who die by suicide have these risk factors, and most people who do have them are not suicidal. Signs include the following:

- Social isolation that may be self-imposed
- Drastic mood swings or overall personality changes
- Neglecting home, finances or pets

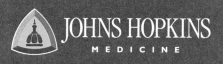

LATEST RESEARCH

Delayed Heart Attack Care for Depression Patients

Patients who visit an emergency department with a heart attack may receive delayed treatment if they've had depression.

In a new study, Canadian researchers pointed to past research that found that patients do more poorly after a heart attack if they have depression. They looked at 6,784 patients who were admitted to 96 Ontario hospitals with a heart attack to see if those with a history of depression were more likely to be considered lower priority when they arrived in the emergency department.

Of those patients, 10 percent of patients had a history of depression. In all, 39 percent were given a low-priority score, compared with just 33 percent of people without a history of depression. Patients with depression were also about three minutes slower to receive an electrocardiogram (a test to check out their heart rhythm) and more than two hours slower to receive percutaneous coronary intervention (a treatment to open up the heart's blood vessels using a balloon inflated through a catheter).

One possibility is that emergency department staff assume that in people with depression, their chest pain or other possible heart attack symptoms may be due to depression or anxiety rather than lack of blood flow to the heart. Further studies are needed to understand all the factors contributing to this delay.

CMAJ: CANADIAN MEDICAL ASSOCIATION JOURNAL
Volume 183, page 663
April 5, 2011

Depression and Diabetes

Why are the two conditions linked, and what can you do to prevent and treat them?

Two of the most common health problems in the United States are depression and diabetes. Nearly 15 million American adults are diagnosed with depression in any given year, and more than 23 million people have diabetes. But depression and diabetes have more in common than just their prevalence—each can increase your risk of having the other.

This link has been demonstrated in several studies. Depression may increase your risk of type 2 diabetes, although the link is not as strong as it is for diabetes increasing the risk of depression. Twenty to 25 percent of people with diabetes are estimated to have clinically significant depression—twice the rate of those without diabetes.

Managing either depression or diabetes can be difficult. Having both can be even more challenging. People with both tend to have more severe symptoms of each disease and require more medical services. Fortunately, treatment is available for both depression and diabetes.

Why depression increases your diabetes risk

Experts still don't fully understand why depression and diabetes are so strongly linked, but a mix of biological and behavioral factors seems to be at work. Factors that may make those with depression more susceptible to type 2 diabetes include:

• **Cortisol.** Also known as the stress hormone, cortisol is involved in blood glucose metabolism and insulin sensitivity. People with depression have high cortisol levels, which are also associated with increased fat deposits in the abdomen—a risk factor for type 2 diabetes.

• **Unhealthy lifestyle choices.** If you are depressed, you may not have the energy or motivation to exercise or eat a healthy diet. You may turn to smoking or other unhealthy behaviors that can increase your risk of diabetes.

Why diabetes can bring on depression

Factors that may cause those with diabetes to experience depression include:

• **Illness burden.** This phrase refers to the psychological impact of a chronic illness—in other words, simply knowing you have diabetes can lead to depression.

• **Diabetes-related stress.** Managing a chronic condition—especially one such as diabetes, which can require significant lifestyle changes—is stressful, and that stress can lead to depression. If you are diagnosed with diabetes, you may feel that you're missing out on things and that spending time with friends and relatives is too complicated because of your dietary restrictions. As a result, you may withdraw from the people and activities that you love, which can put you at risk for depression.

Why having both is so serious

If you already have diabetes, depression can undermine your ability to manage your blood glucose levels. You may not have the energy to exercise, neglect to take your medications properly or forget to test your blood glucose levels regularly—increasing your risk of long-term diabetes complications.

Having both depression and diabetes has been linked to a higher risk of cardiovascular disease and death. A 2011 research trial looked at the mortality risk in older women with depression and diabetes. Participants included 78,282 female nurses who were between ages 54 and 79 in 2000 and completed health questionnaires every two years through 2006.

Compared with participants who had neither, those who had both depression and diabetes were more than two times as likely to die of any cause and almost three times more likely to die of cardiovascular disease. And the more severe the diabetes combined with depression, the greater the risk. Those who were depressed and had been living with diabetes for more than 10 years were more than three times as likely to die of cardiovascular disease, and those who required insulin therapy were nearly five times as likely to suffer a cardiovascular-related death. This research is significant because most studies on depression and diabetes have been conducted in men, who are less likely than women to have depression.

Another study, which involved both men and women, found that people with type 2 diabetes and major depression are at greater risk not only for cardiovascular disease but also for other life-threatening diabetes complications. Published in *Diabetes Care* in 2010, the study involved more than 4,600 people with diabetes living in Washington state. Five years after

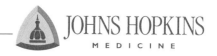

their initial interview, participants with depression had a 36 percent greater risk of microvascular complications, such as blindness and end-stage kidney disease, and a 25 percent higher risk of macrovascular diabetes complications, such as heart attack and stroke.

The good news

While depression may increase your diabetes risk, lifestyle factors remain a more significant influence and can counteract that risk. A *Journal of the American Medical Association (JAMA)* study backs this up: Individuals with depression were found to be 42 percent more likely to develop type 2 diabetes in three years than people who were not depressed—but the increased risk was no longer statistically significant after factoring in for healthy lifestyle (diet, physical activity, smoking status and alcohol use). So if you have depression, adopting or maintaining healthy habits may keep diabetes at bay.

As for depression that was likely brought on by diabetes, standard treatments for depression, such as antidepressants, psychotherapy and exercise, can help. Although exercise alone probably won't be enough to fix either condition completely, it can help improve both mood and blood glucose levels.

Psychotherapy works well for mild to moderate depression and has been shown to have a positive effect on blood glucose levels as well. For moderate to severe depression, antidepressants may work more quickly than psychotherapy, although a combination of the two is most often best. Your

---

Diabetes: What You Need to Know

Diabetes is a chronic disease in which high levels of glucose (sugar) build up in the bloodstream due to insufficient production of insulin by the pancreas, the body's resistance to insulin or a combination of both.

Type 1 diabetes usually develops before age 30 and tends to come on suddenly in normal-weight people. Symptoms include excessive thirst, frequent urination and weight loss.

Type 2 diabetes accounts for 90 to 95 percent of diabetes cases and usually starts later in life in overweight people. It often develops gradually over many years, and the initial symptoms may be almost unnoticeable. In fact, many people find out that they have type 2 diabetes when a routine laboratory test shows high blood glucose levels. As glucose levels continue to increase, most people develop the classic initial symptoms of type 1 diabetes.

Other symptoms of type 2 diabetes include:
• Blurred vision
• Weakness and fatigue
• Recurrent yeast infections
• Infections of the skin and gums

In some people, peripheral neuropathy (nerve damage in the hands or feet) or coronary heart disease are among the first indicators of diabetes. These complications can be controlled but cannot be cured once they develop. That's why the American Diabetes Association recommends that all people age 45 and older be screened for the disease every three years. The association recommends more frequent screening—every one to two years—for people who have a parent or sibling with diabetes, levels of beneficial high density lipoprotein (HDL) cholesterol below 40 mg/dL, triglyceride levels above 150 mg/dL or prediabetes (a fasting blood glucose level of 100 to 125 mg/dL). The ADA also recommends more frequent screenings for those who were diagnosed with diabetes during pregnancy or who delivered a baby weighing more than 9 lbs.

---

primary care physician or a psychiatrist can determine which medication is best for you. (For more information on antidepressants, see pages 19-33.) If you have diabetes, be sure to ask about side effects that could impact your disease, such as weight gain or any effects the drug may have on your blood glucose level. To find a mental health professional with experience treating individuals with diabetes, contact your local chapter of the American Diabetes Association (www.diabetes.org). They may be able to refer you to mental health professionals in your area. ∎

- Recent psychological trauma, such as a divorce, death of a loved one or job loss (which may trigger suicidal thinking in an already depressed person)
- Exaggerated complaints of aches or pains
- Giving away cherished belongings to loved ones or putting one's affairs in order
- Sudden calm or cheerfulness after a period of depression
- Frequent use of alcohol or other drugs
- Buying a gun
- Verbal threats of suicide or statements that suggest a desire to die
- Family history of suicide or previous suicide attempts

Natural History and Prognosis of Mood Disorders

Mood disorders most often surface around the age of 30 but they can occur at any age. An accurate diagnosis is often delayed because symptoms are typically not recognized as being related to an illness. Instead, they are thought to be a reaction to life circumstances.

Depression

An untreated episode of major depression usually lasts eight to nine months. This period can be shortened considerably with proper diagnosis and treatment. Most people with depression have their first episode before age 40, and most will have more than one episode in their lifetime. Relapse rates are lower in people who continue with treatment when they are feeling well. Approximately 15 percent of depressed people have a chronic form of depression that is resistant to current treatments.

Alcoholism or other drug use can make recovery from depression (and bipolar disorder) more difficult. A recent study compared 176 men and women who fit the criteria for both alcoholism and major depression with 412 people who had major depression alone. Those who had never been alcoholics or who no longer drank were twice as likely to recover from an episode of major depression than those who were still drinking. Unfortunately, many depressed people slow their recovery by attempting to self-medicate with alcohol.

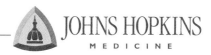

Bipolar Disorder

Bipolar disorder usually begins at an earlier age than depression and can even occur in childhood. But it is also an unpredictable disease that can emerge later in life. In one large study of people treated at Veterans Affairs hospitals, 25 percent of the more than 65,000 people with bipolar disorder treated during one year were age 60 or older. And in this over-60 age group, approximately 6 percent had new-onset disease.

In a second study, about 10 percent of 1,157 people between the ages of 18 and 70 treated in an urban primary care clinic screened positive for bipolar disorder. Of those, 41 percent reported first being affected at age 40 or older. Another study suggests that 10 percent of new cases occur after age 50.

Overall, men and women are equally likely to suffer from bipolar disorder, but women may be more likely to experience the late-onset form. A study of 48 older adults with bipolar disorder showed that women were almost three times as likely to be in the late-onset group.

About two-thirds of people with bipolar disorder who recover completely from an acute episode have recurrent bouts of either depression or mania. Half of these recurrences tend to be manic, even when the first episode is depression. Although the average number of recurrences is four, this number can vary significantly from person to person. The episodes can be separated by weeks, months or years. Over time, recurrences tend to happen more frequently, and they may become more severe.

Some people with bipolar disorder can cycle between depressive and manic episodes as often as four times a year. This is known as rapid cycling. There is tremendous variability in the course of the condition, with some people experiencing full recovery between episodes and others experiencing chronic (ongoing) symptoms.

Treatment of Mood Disorders

In treating depression, doctors have three goals. The first is to relieve the symptoms of depression, the second is to restore the person's ability to function socially and in the workplace, and the final goal is to reduce the likelihood of a recurrence.

The goals for bipolar disorder are somewhat different because the disease is usually more challenging to treat. Doctors primarily strive to reduce the frequency and severity—and the social and psychological impact—of episodes. Improving social and mental functioning between episodes is the other major goal of treatment.

When a person seeks treatment for a mood disorder, the first step is a complete evaluation, which includes a detailed psychiatric and medical history, and a mental status examination. Because treatment varies considerably based on the diagnosis, it is crucial to have this comprehensive assessment.

Treatment goals for depression and bipolar disorder are met in three stages—acute, continuation and maintenance. During *acute treatment*, the focus is on immediately relieving symptoms and restoring the person's ability to function. Once symptoms respond to acute treatment, *continuation treatment* begins; the focus here is on preventing a relapse. If a person has no symptoms for four to nine months after an episode, he or she is considered recovered. At this point, *maintenance treatment* begins, with the goal of preventing a new episode. Maintenance treatment can last from one year to a lifetime, depending on the individual.

Depression recurs in about half of cases within two years of ending treatment, so timing must be considered carefully when stopping medications. The longer a person remains on treatment, the smaller the likelihood of relapse. The decision to try tapering off medications for bipolar disorder is more complicated because it involves the risk of recurrent manic and depressive episodes and, especially, the risk of suicide.

The main treatment options for dealing with depression and bipolar disorder are medications, psychotherapy, electroconvulsive therapy (sometimes informally referred to as shock therapy), or any combination of these. Light therapy is often used to treat SAD. In addition, exercise, getting enough sleep and eating a healthy diet play a role in improving mood and self-image.

These days, medications are often the recommended initial treatment choice for people with mild-to-moderate depression or severe major depression. Any given antidepressant has up to a 70 percent chance of working in a particular person. It is important to start treatment as early as possible, as these disorders become more difficult to treat the longer they last. Because response to any particular treatment varies from one person to another, an individual who does not improve with the initial treatment may respond to a different one.

In fact, that's the important lesson to be learned from a large, six-year multicenter study called the Sequenced Treatment Alternatives to Relieve Depression, or STAR*D, trial which looked at the use of popular antidepressants in people with chronic depression (lasting,

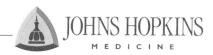

in some cases, 15 to 16 years). This study found that systematically trying different doses of antidepressant medications, maintaining a longer duration of therapy, trying a different drug altogether or combining medications can lead to a remission in symptoms for many severely depressed, treatment-resistant patients.

Like antidepressant medications, psychotherapy alone also can work to relieve depression—usually with fewer side effects. While it requires more time than antidepressant therapy to reduce symptoms, its positive effects may last longer than medication. Psychotherapy alone is often recommended as an initial treatment option for people with mild-to-moderate depression.

Severe cases of depression are best treated with medication. In the most extreme cases, electroconvulsive therapy (ECT) may be recommended. Up to 90 percent of extremely depressed people improve with ECT when it is used as a first-line treatment. However, the therapy is usually used only after other therapies have failed. When used as a last resort, the response rate drops to 50 to 60 percent (see "ECT: Effective Treatment for Severe Depression" on pages 48-49).

Combination therapy (medication plus psychotherapy) has been shown in some research studies to be more effective than either therapy alone for mild-to-moderate depression. This option may be beneficial if either treatment alone produces only partial results, if depression is chronic, or if the person is facing multiple challenges that are best treated by different means, such as medication for depressive symptoms and psychotherapy for job-related problems. Recent research suggests that combination therapy may prevent or delay relapses and recurrences of depression.

Treatment of Depression with Medications

Today, physicians can choose from a wide range of antidepressant medications (see the drug chart on pages 24-25). These include selective serotonin reuptake inhibitors (SSRIs), tricyclics, tetracyclics, dopamine reuptake inhibitors, serotonin and norepinephrine reuptake inhibitors, monoamine oxidase (MAO) inhibitors and a new category, SSRI/5-HT1A receptor partial agonist.

There are several advantages to treating depression with antidepressant medications:

- They are effective against mild, moderate and severe forms of major depression.
- People usually respond more quickly to medications than to psychotherapy.

- They are easy to administer.
- They are not addictive and, when properly used, are usually quite safe.
- They can be used in combination with psychotherapy.

The disadvantages are:

- Medication therapy can cause unwanted side effects.
- It requires strict adherence to a medication schedule and repeated visits to your doctor to monitor response.
- It may take some time—and some tinkering—to find the right medication at the right dose.

Because of these factors, many people do not have an adequate trial of a therapeutic dose for a sufficient period of time. Older individuals and those with chronic illnesses are more susceptible to the adverse effects of antidepressants.

Researchers believe that antidepressants work by affecting levels of neurotransmitters—chemical messengers in the brain that facilitate communication between nerve cells. However, physicians cannot predetermine which medication will be the most effective in any particular individual. Drug selection relies largely on a process of educated guesses, although most people do have some positive response to the first antidepressant they try.

Choosing a medication

For a person with a first-time episode of moderate-to-severe depression and no other psychological symptoms or medical conditions, the choice of medication is generally based on avoidance of side effects. For example, the tricyclic antidepressant amitriptyline can lower blood pressure and cause drowsiness and confusion—side effects that are especially troublesome for older people. The drug nortriptyline (Aventyl, Pamelor) is less likely to cause these side effects.

Family history can also help predict which drugs are most likely to be effective, as well as which ones are most likely to cause side effects. In addition, older people are typically started on lower doses than younger people to reduce the risk of side effects.

By themselves, antidepressant medications usually produce a significant improvement by four to eight weeks, although it may take up to 12 weeks to see the full benefit. If a person's depression responds fully to medication after this period, treatment moves on to the continuation phase, which lasts for six months to one year at the same dosage level. People who have had three or more prior major depressive episodes or who have chronic major depression

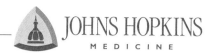

should continue on to a maintenance phase (continuation at the same dosage level). Those who have improved somewhat but still have a few symptoms after six weeks should be reassessed six weeks later (many are likely to improve further during this time). At the reassessment, the physician may adjust the dosage to improve response.

When a drug does not work, a doctor may prescribe an antidepressant from a different class of medications, because drugs in the same class tend to work similarly. When a drug from one class is producing good results but causes unacceptable side effects, switching to a different drug within the same class can often help.

In 20 to 50 percent of people, adding the drug lithium can help boost the effect of an antidepressant. However, the addition of lithium increases the risk of side effects and adverse drug interactions, requiring close monitoring by a physician.

If maintenance treatment is no longer needed, drugs are discontinued slowly over a period of one to three weeks to avoid withdrawal symptoms. Relapses are most common during the first two months after a person stops taking an antidepressant. It is therefore important for individuals to remain in contact with their physicians during this period. Should a relapse occur, the same drug that was used successfully the first time often proves effective again.

Suicide and medication

All antidepressants must be used with caution if a person is suicidal. When this is the case, the person will need to see his or her doctor for frequent follow-up visits and will receive a prescription for a relatively small number of pills at a time to determine their effectiveness. Suicide attempts or suicidal thoughts are common symptoms of depression, and the risk of suicide may increase as depression begins to respond to treatment because the person might regain just enough energy and motivation to follow through on a suicidal urge.

In 2004, a federal panel of drug experts said that antidepressants could increase the risk of suicide in children and teenagers. Later that year, the Food and Drug Administration (FDA) required the makers of antidepressants to add a black box warning to that effect to the drug labels of these medications. In 2005, the agency issued a public health advisory stating that suicidal thoughts and behaviors may also increase among adults on antidepressants. And a 2010 study found that suicide risk is the same for all antidepressants. The risk of suicide is higher at the start of drug therapy and when the dosage is changed, according to the FDA.

Antidepressants are the fourth leading cause of drug overdose and the third leading cause of drug-related death when taken improperly. Tricyclics such as amitriptyline are the most common cause of death from an antidepressant overdose. In addition, when a person with latent bipolar disorder starts taking antidepressants, manic symptoms may develop and require treatment.

Although up to 70 percent of people with depression respond positively to antidepressants—and some studies suggest that use of antidepressants, particularly newer SSRIs, decreases the risk of suicide—it is true that some people might have responded just as well to a placebo. But whether a person responds to an antidepressant because of the action of the medication or the placebo effect, or possibly a combination of the two, the fact remains that antidepressants provide real relief to many people. Moreover, because studies of the placebo effect have only followed people for a limited period of time, there are no data showing whether the placebo effect can be sustained in the long term. By contrast, there are data showing that the positive effects of medication are sustained long term.

When it comes to the length of treatment for depression, there is no "one size fits all." However, recent evidence shows that many people require a year or more of antidepressant therapy to treat a major depressive episode adequately. (This includes roughly three months of acute treatment to significantly improve depressive symptoms and an additional six months to a year of continuation/maintenance treatment.) People with severe or recurring depression and older adults may require much longer maintenance therapy.

Selective serotonin reuptake inhibitors (SSRIs)
Low amounts of the neurotransmitter serotonin have been linked to depression. SSRIs such as citalopram (Celexa), escitalopram (Lexapro), fluoxetine (Prozac), fluvoxamine (Luvox), paroxetine (Paxil) and sertraline (Zoloft) increase levels of serotonin in the brain. All of the SSRIs are equally effective and have similar rates and types of side effects, although it is possible that an individual might respond better or experience fewer side effects with a particular SSRI. Side effects are not always a reason to change medications. For example, Paxil can produce a sedative effect in some people, but this may benefit people who suffer from both anxiety and depression.

Because the side effects of SSRIs are milder than those of most

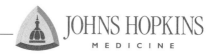

other antidepressants, most doctors consider them the first-line drug treatment for depression. Studies have demonstrated that SSRIs are as effective as tricyclics. About half of those who take an SSRI see their symptoms of depression lift completely. Advantages of SSRIs over other antidepressants, such as tricyclics, include a lower risk of fatal overdoses and serious heart rhythm disturbances in people with heart disease. SSRIs are also effective against dysthymia (chronic low-grade depression).

Side effects. SSRIs can produce side effects such as anxiety, nervousness, insomnia, drowsiness and nausea. Another troublesome side effect is sexual dysfunction—diminished sexual desire, changes in the sensations of arousal or disturbances in the ability to achieve orgasm—which may occur in about 37 percent of both men and women taking these drugs. Sexual side effects usually develop within the first week of starting an SSRI, though they may arise more slowly as blood levels of the medication build up. Strategies to alleviate sexual dysfunction include switching to a medication with a low rate of sexual side effects (such as the dopamine reuptake inhibitor bupropion [Wellbutrin]), waiting to see if sexual side effects abate, changing the time when you take the medication (possibly to nighttime), reducing the dosage, taking drug holidays (for example, not taking the medication on the weekend) or adding an erectile dysfunction drug like sildenafil (Viagra). If you experience worrisome symptoms, do not make any changes in your drug regimen on your own—be sure to consult your doctor first.

Recently, it was recognized that SSRIs may produce neurological side effects—symptoms like those of Parkinson's disease, such as impaired muscle tone, tremors, spasms or feelings of restlessness. These symptoms can become so severe that sitting still becomes impossible. Fortunately, they are rare. In one study, they occurred in only 0.3 percent of people. By comparison, the most common side effects of Prozac—agitation and anxiety—occurred in twice as many people, although they were still relatively uncommon. If you experience any of these symptoms, contact your doctor before you stop taking your medication.

In addition, people taking a combination of drugs that raise the level of serotonin in the body can develop a disorder called serotonin syndrome. The most common causes are taking an SSRI at the same time as a monoamine oxidase (MAO) inhibitor or a triptan migraine drug (for example, frovatriptan [Frova], rizatriptan [Maxalt], sumatriptan [Imitrex] and others). The syndrome is characterized by altered mental status, neuromuscular abnormalities and

Antidepressant Drugs 2012*

Drug type: Brand (generic)	Typical daily dosage†	How they appear to work
Selective serotonin reuptake inhibitors (SSRIs)		
Celexa (citalopram‡)	20-40 mg	Block the reabsorption and inactivation of the neurotransmitter serotonin. This increases the availability of serotonin to carry messages between nerve cells.
Lexapro (escitalopram)	10-20 mg	
Luvox (fluvoxamine‡)	50-300 mg	
Luvox CR (fluvoxamine, controlled-release)	100-300 mg	
Paxil (paroxetine‡)	20-50 mg	
Paxil CR (paroxetine, controlled-release‡)	12.5-62.5 mg	
Prozac (fluoxetine‡)	20-80 mg	
Prozac Weekly (fluoxetine)	90 mg	
Zoloft (sertraline‡)	50-200 mg	
Serotonin and norepinephrine reuptake inhibitors (SNRIs)		
Cymbalta (duloxetine)	40-60 mg	Block the reabsorption of serotonin and norepinephrine, increasing the availability of these neurotransmitters in the brain.
Effexor (venlafaxine‡)	75-375 mg	
Effexor XR (venlafaxine, extended-release)	37.5-225 mg	
Oleptro (trazodone§)	150-400 mg	
Pristiq (desvenlafaxine)	50 mg	
Dopamine reuptake inhibitors		
Wellbutrin (bupropion‡)	200-450 mg	Block the reabsorption of the neurotransmitter dopamine, increasing its availability in the brain.
Wellbutrin SR (bupropion, sustained-release‡)	150-400 mg	
Wellbutrin XL (bupropion, extended-release‡)	150-450 mg	
Tricyclics		
Elavil (amitriptyline)	50-200 mg	Block the reabsorption of the neurotransmitters serotonin, norepinephrine and, to a lesser extent, dopamine, increasing their availability in the brain.
Aventyl (nortriptyline‡)	75-150 mg	
Norpramin (desipramine‡)	100-300 mg	
Pamelor (nortriptyline‡)	75-150 mg	
Silenor (doxepin‡)	25-300 mg	
Surmontil (trimipramine‡)	50-200 mg	
Tofranil (imipramine‡)	75-200 mg	
Vivactil (protriptyline‡)	15-60 mg	

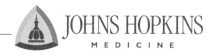

Precautions	Common side effects
Do not take with monoamine oxidase (MAO) inhibitors, triptans, or St. John's wort. If discontinuing use, reduce dosage gradually to prevent withdrawal symptoms. The development of a skin rash can be the sign of a serious medical problem; see a doctor immediately. *Celexa only*: This drug should no longer be used at doses greater than 40 mg a day due to risk of causing abnormal changes in the electrical activity of the heart.	Anxiety, nervousness, insomnia, drowsiness, weakness, headache, diarrhea, increased sweating, nausea, impaired sexual function, weight gain. Side effects appear to be lesser with Lexapro.
Do not take with MAO inhibitors or triptans. If discontinuing use, reduce dosage gradually to prevent withdrawal symptoms. Effexor and Pristiq may increase blood pressure and/or cholesterol levels, especially at high doses; regular blood pressure and cholesterol monitoring is advised. Effexor may cause abnormal bleeding, especially in people taking aspirin, nonsteroidal anti-inflammatory drugs (NSAIDs), warfarin or other anticoagulants.	Nausea, weakness, sweating, insomnia, drowsiness, dry mouth, dizziness, constipation, nervousness, impaired sexual function, appetite loss.
Do not take if you have seizures or an eating disorder, are using MAO inhibitors or are using another product that contains bupropion (such as the smoking-cessation drug Zyban). Wellbutrin (not SR or XL) must be given in divided doses at least 8 hours apart, with no single dose exceeding 150 mg.	Appetite and weight loss, dry mouth, rash, sweating, ears ringing, stomach pain, agitation, anxiety, dizziness, trouble sleeping, muscle pain, nausea, fast heartbeat, sore throat, increased urination. Greater risk of seizures at higher doses. Low risk of sexual side effects and weight gain.
Do not take with MAO inhibitors. Do not stop treatment abruptly. It is not advisable to take most tricyclic antidepressants if you have seizures, a heart disorder or glaucoma, or if you use alcohol excessively.	Dizziness on standing, drowsiness, weakness, headache, dry mouth, blurred vision, constipation, nausea, difficulty urinating, increased appetite (which may include a craving for sweets), impaired sexual function, increased heart rate. Skin is more sensitive to sunlight, which may result in itching, redness, discoloration of skin.

* This list represents the most commonly prescribed antidepressants.

† These dosages represent an average range for the treatment of depression and may differ from the dosage prescribed by your doctor. The precise effective dosage varies from person to person and depends on many factors. Do not make any change to your medication without consulting your doctor. *Starting dosages tend to be lower for older adults.*

‡ Generic version available at lower cost.

§ Generic only available.

continued on the next page

Antidepressant Drugs 2012 * (continued)

Drug type: Brand (generic)	Typical daily dosage[†]	How they appear to work
Tetracyclics		
Ludiomil (maprotiline)	75-200 mg	Block the reabsorption of serotonin and norepinephrine, increasing the availability of these neurotransmitters.
Remeron (mirtazapine[‡])	15-45 mg	
Remeron SolTab (mirtazapine[‡])	15-45 mg	
Monoamine oxidase (MAO) inhibitors		
Emsam skin patch (selegiline)	6-12 mg	Block the action of MAO, an enzyme that inactivates the neurotransmitters serotonin, norepinephrine and dopamine. MAO inhibitors thereby increase levels of these neurotransmitters, increasing their availability for carrying messages between neurons.
Marplan (isocarboxazid[‡])	10-60 mg	
Nardil (phenelzine[‡])	45-90 mg	
Parnate (tranylcypromine[‡])	10-30 mg	
Atypical neuroleptic/selective serotonin reuptake inhibitor		
Symbyax (olanzapine/fluoxetine)	3/25-12/50 mg	Increases the availability of the neurotransmitters serotonin, norepinephrine and dopamine to treat depression.
SSRI/5-HT 1A receptor partial agonist		
Viibryd (vilazodone)	40 mg	Blocks the reabsorption of the neurotransmitter serotonin, increasing the availability of serotonin to carry messages between nerve cells. The mechanism of its effect on 5-HT 1A receptors is not fully understood.

[*] This list represents the most commonly prescribed antidepressants.

[†] These dosages represent an average range for the treatment of depression and may differ from the dosage prescribed by your doctor. The precise effective dosage varies from patient to patient and depends on many factors. Do not make any change to your medication without consulting your doctor. *Starting dosages tend to be lower for older adults.*

[‡] Generic version available at lower cost.

[§] Generic only available.

dysfunction of the autonomic nervous system, which controls involuntary reflexes that affect breathing, heart rate, blood pressure and the digestive tract. Tricyclic antidepressants may also contribute to serotonin syndrome.

SSRIs can increase the risk of gastrointestinal bleeding, particularly when taken with nonsteroidal anti-inflammatory drugs (NSAIDs), such as aspirin, according to a recent Danish study. This increased risk of bleeding means blood is less likely to clot, an effect that may be beneficial to certain people at risk for heart attacks and ischemic

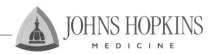

Precautions	Common side effects
Do not take with MAO inhibitors. Caution advised with use of Remeron in the elderly because of delayed metabolism and clearance of the drug, which may increase the risk of adverse events.	Sleepiness, nausea, increased appetite, weight gain, dizziness, blurred vision, weakness, dry mouth, headache, constipation, shakiness, nervousness.
Foods containing tyramine (see page 31) should be avoided because they may cause a sudden, severe rise in blood pressure (hypertensive crisis), which can be fatal. There are no dietary restrictions with the 6-mg Emsam skin patch, as it does not interfere with the breakdown of tyramine in the digestive tract. (Restrictions do apply for the higher-dose patches.) MAO inhibitors may interact dangerously with numerous drugs, including other antidepressants and cold medications.	Dizziness, lightheadedness (especially in older persons), drowsiness, headache, dry mouth, constipation, nausea, insomnia, decreased sexual function, weight gain. Patch can cause skin irritation.
Atypical neuroleptics increase the risk of death in elderly patients with dementia. See a doctor immediately if you experience signs of neuroleptic malignant syndrome (characterized by muscle stiffness or spasms, high fever, and confusion or disorientation) or infection (fever, chills, sweating and fatigue).	Weight gain, sleepiness, increased appetite, weakness, swelling in legs and arms, tremors, sore throat, difficulty concentrating.
Do not take with MAO inhibitors. If discontinuing use, reduce dosage gradually to prevent withdrawal symptoms.	Diarrhea, nausea, insomnia, vomiting.

strokes—conditions caused by blood clotting. Another study found that depressed heart patients treated with the SSRI Zoloft showed significant reductions in the level of clotting factors in their blood compared with those receiving a placebo. However, in people already taking an anticoagulant to prevent or treat blood clots, an SSRI may increase the risk of gastrointestinal bleeding.

A recent Canadian study found that SSRIs may increase the risk of fractures in older adults, possibly by compromising bone quality and strength as well as by increasing the chance of falling.

Although side effects tend to be similar among SSRIs, Luvox and Paxil may be more likely to cause nausea, and diarrhea is more common with Zoloft. Because Prozac may take several days to clear from the body, interactions with other drugs are more likely to occur. One advantage of Prozac, however, is that it is now available in a once-a-week capsule.

SSRI withdrawal. SSRIs are not addictive in the conventional medical use of the word, but suddenly discontinuing their use after taking them for more than six weeks is known to produce both physical and psychological withdrawal symptoms.

About one-quarter of people who abruptly stop taking an SSRI experience dizziness, nausea, lethargy and headache. Other symptoms include irritability, nervousness, crying spells, flu-like symptoms (body aches, chills and fatigue), and shooting pains in and around the head.

SSRI withdrawal—also called SSRI discontinuation syndrome—is not dangerous, but it can be distressing. Fortunately, it is usually mild, commences within one week of stopping treatment and resolves within three weeks.

To minimize SSRI discontinuation syndrome, doses of SSRIs (like other antidepressants) should be reduced gradually.

SSRI/5-HT1A receptor partial agonist

In 2011, the FDA approved a new medication for major depressive disorder, vilazodone (Viibryd), which is the first in a new class of antidepressant, SSRI/5-HT1A receptor partial agonist. Viibryd works partly in the same way as SSRIs by blocking the reabsorption of serotonin and increasing its availability to carry messages between nerve cells. Viibryd also works on 5-HT1A receptors, although the way in which it does is not fully understood. Viibryd should not be taken in conjunction with MAO inhibitors. Common side effects include diarrhea, nausea, vomiting and insomnia. When discontinuing treatment with Viibryd, it should be done gradually (as with SSRIs) to avoid possible withdrawal symptoms, such as dizziness, headache, irritability and flu-like symptoms.

Tricyclics

Tricyclics—such as amitriptyline (Elavil), desipramine (Norpramin), doxepin (Silenor), imipramine (Tofranil), nortriptyline (Aventyl, Pamelor), protriptyline (Vivactil) and trimipramine (Surmontil)—are named for their chemical structure. These drugs raise brain concentrations of the neurotransmitters norepinephrine, serotonin

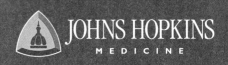

and, to a lesser extent, dopamine, by blocking reabsorption of these chemical messengers by the nerve cells that release them. Tricyclics are used mainly to treat moderate-to-severe depression and have proven less effective for chronic low-grade depression. About 60 percent of people who take tricyclics experience significant improvement within four to six weeks. Each of the tricyclics is believed to be equally effective, but side effects may differ.

When a person begins tricyclic therapy, he or she is given a small dose and is carefully monitored for side effects. The dose is often raised over several weeks because a gradual increase may be less likely to lead to side effects. Side effects also tend to diminish with continued use. For older people, dosages are usually 30 to 50 percent lower than those indicated in the chart on pages 24-27. When the proper dosage is established, tricyclics can be taken at bedtime so that any resulting drowsiness occurs before sleep rather than during the day.

Although a positive response to tricyclics typically appears within four to six weeks, doctors recommend taking the medication for six to eight weeks at full dosage to assess the effects. During this time, blood tests may be ordered to make sure that the drug level is high enough to exert a therapeutic effect but not so high as to be toxic. If a person's depression does not improve while taking a tricyclic, it may be that the drug is not effective for that person or that he or she is not taking the drug as prescribed. About one-third of people stop taking tricyclics because of side effects, and about two-thirds of older people miss 25 to 50 percent of their doses. Poor compliance leads to fluctuating blood levels of the drug and, consequently, a poor response. Therefore, it is important to tell your doctor about unpleasant side effects instead of just stopping your medication.

Side effects. The most prominent side effects of tricyclics are postural hypotension (dizziness on standing due to a drop in blood pressure), drowsiness, weakness, headache, dry mouth, blurred vision, constipation, nausea and difficulty urinating. Many of these side effects can be managed, however. Drowsiness can be remedied by taking the dose before bedtime (if your doctor approves). Postural hypotension, which can lead to falls and broken bones in older people, can be reduced by standing up slowly after sitting or lying down and waiting 30 seconds before trying to walk. Pilocarpine (Pilocar) eyedrops may alleviate blurred vision. Chewing sugar-free gum or candy will help dry mouth. (Be sure to mention dry mouth to your dentist—a lack of saliva can lead to an increase in cavities and oral infections.) Bethanechol (Duvoid, Urabeth,

Urecholine) may be prescribed to counteract problems with urination. And constipation can be managed by consuming foods high in fiber and drinking at least eight glasses of water or juice a day. Amitriptyline and Tofranil are more likely than other tricyclics to cause side effects in older people.

People who should not take tricyclics. Tricyclics are not given to people with closed-angle glaucoma and should be used with caution in men who have symptoms of benign prostatic hyperplasia (enlarged prostate), as they may lose the ability to urinate. This medical emergency must be treated with catheterization. Tricyclics can also magnify the depressive effects of alcohol and benzodiazepines. The combination of tricyclics with antihistamines can lead to severe constipation, impacted stools or difficulty urinating, particularly in older adults. In addition, tricyclics (and SSRIs) should not be mixed with the drug selegiline (Eldepryl), which is used to treat Parkinson's disease. Although rare, an interaction between these drugs may cause high fever, tremors, agitation, restlessness or, in some cases, death. Other symptoms resulting from such drug combinations may include fainting, profuse sweating, seizures, behavioral changes and stiffened muscles.

Tricyclics are not currently recommended for use in most people with coronary heart disease (CHD) because they can cause life-threatening ventricular fibrillation (abnormal rhythm in the heart's lower chambers) in these individuals. Despite the heart risks of tricyclics, they are still used to treat depression because they are sometimes the only effective antidepressants for severely depressed older people.

An older person with mild-to-moderate depression and severe CHD may first be given a medication from another drug class (an SSRI, such as Luvox, Celexa, Lexapro, Prozac, Paxil or Zoloft, or the dopamine reuptake inhibitor Wellbutrin). If the individual does not respond to these drugs, a tricyclic would then be tried. Because the risk of ventricular fibrillation from tricyclics increases with the severity of CHD, the doctor must weigh the severity of the depression against the potential danger to the heart.

Tetracyclics
The action, efficacy and side effects of drugs like maprotiline and mirtazapine (Remeron) are similar to those of the tricyclics. However, maprotiline is more likely to cause seizures than most other antidepressants. A version of Remeron is available that dissolves on the tongue and does not need to be chewed or swallowed whole.

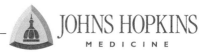

Dopamine reuptake inhibitors

Wellbutrin decreases the reuptake of dopamine, a neurotransmitter and a precursor of other neurotransmitters. This drug causes less drowsiness and fewer side effects than the tricyclics (especially fewer sexual side effects), but on rare occasions it can cause seizures, particularly at higher doses. Wellbutrin XL is the first drug approved to prevent major depressive episodes in people with seasonal affective disorder (SAD).

Serotonin and norepinephrine reuptake inhibitors

Medications like desvenlafaxine (Pristiq), duloxetine (Cymbalta), trazodone (Oleptro) and venlafaxine (Effexor) are serotonin and norepinephrine reuptake inhibitors (SNRIs). These medications work by raising brain concentrations of the neurotransmitters serotonin and norepinephrine. SNRIs are often the most effective drugs for older people. Possible side effects include nausea, weakness, sweating, insomnia, drowsiness, dry mouth, dizziness and constipation. Effexor may increase blood pressure and cholesterol levels in some people, so monitoring blood pressure and cholesterol is important for anyone taking this drug. Cymbalta, Effexor and Pristiq taken in combination with triptan migraine medications may result in serotonin syndrome.

Monoamine oxidase (MAO) inhibitors

MAO inhibitors such as phenelzine (Nardil) and tranylcypromine (Parnate) increase brain levels of norepinephrine, serotonin and dopamine by blocking the action of the enzyme MAO, which normally inactivates these three neurotransmitters. MAO inhibitors are effective in many depressed people, especially those whose depression is accompanied by marked anxiety, panic attacks, heightened appetite or excessive sleeping.

People who should not take MAO inhibitors. MAO inhibitors can cause some of the same side effects as the tricyclics; side effects can be reduced in similar ways (see "Side effects" on page 29). But there are some individuals for whom MAO inhibitors pose greater risks. If you are a heavy drinker, have heart failure or severely impaired liver or kidney function, or take multiple medications for high blood pressure, you should not take an MAO inhibitor. In addition, MAO inhibitors can cause a sudden, extreme elevation in blood pressure (known as a hypertensive crisis) when people using them take certain drugs or consume foods or beverages containing tyramine. (Tyramine is found in nasal decongestants, cold or allergy medicines, very ripe bananas, beer and aged or smoked meats, among other things.) People taking an MAO inhibitor must get a complete list of restricted foods and drugs from their doctor.

Normally, the enzyme MAO breaks down any tyramine consumed in the diet, preventing its blood pressure-raising effect. This protective mechanism is disabled by MAO inhibitors, which block the action of MAO in the liver and intestine, allowing tyramine levels to rise and increase blood pressure. Symptoms of a hypertensive crisis include severe chest pain, excruciating headache, sweating, clammy skin, nausea and vomiting. Immediate treatment with blood pressure-lowering drugs is essential. Because of this risk and the dietary restrictions, MAO inhibitors are now only used as second-line drugs for the treatment of depression, despite their proven efficacy.

A skin patch of the MAO inhibitor Emsam is now available. At the lowest dose, Emsam does not interfere with the breakdown of tyramine in the digestive tract and can therefore be used without dietary restrictions.

Atypical neuroleptic/selective serotonin reuptake inhibitor

Symbyax, a combination of an atypical neuroleptic (olanzapine) used for bipolar disorder plus an SSRI (fluoxetine), treats depression in people who have not responded to two other antidepressants. Like all neuroleptics, Symbyax increases the risk of death in elderly people with dementia. Symbyax is also associated with a risk of neuroleptic malignant syndrome (see the chart on page 26).

Atypical neuroleptics as adjuncts to antidepressants

Sometimes even after trying several different antidepressants, symptoms of depression remain. In this case, adding an atypical neuroleptic such as aripiprazole (Abilify) or risperidone (Risperdal) to a patient's current medication often provides relief. These medications are approved by the FDA to treat symptoms of bipolar disorder and schizophrenia as well as depression in combination with an antidepressant.

Side effects of neuroleptics include nausea, vomiting, constipation, headache, dizziness, an inner sense of restlessness or need to move (akathisia), anxiety and insomnia. There is also the risk of more serious side effects including a condition called tardive dyskinesia, which causes abnormal or uncontrollable movements of the face, tongue or other parts of the body, and neuroleptic malignant syndrome, which may cause severe muscle stiffness, fever, severe tiredness or weakness.

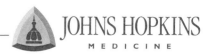

Elderly people with dementia who take neuroleptics are at increased risk of sudden cardiac death. Ask your health-care provider about this and other risks if he or she suggests you take a neuroleptic.

Treatment in older adults

Older people are more susceptible to adverse effects than younger people, so drug therapy must be approached carefully. Smaller dosages as well as closer monitoring for toxic reactions are often required, and ensuring that the medications are being taken as prescribed may be an issue. Drug interactions are a concern, as the elderly use prescription drugs more than the general population. Treatment can also be difficult in reluctant individuals and in those lacking a social support system to help them with practical considerations, such as costs and transportation for visits to a doctor.

Despite all of these obstacles, older people usually respond well to treatment for depression; even partial success can lead to improved quality of life and productivity. Some studies even suggest that treatment with medications is more effective in older individuals than in younger ones.

Alternative treatments

Many people are curious about alternative treatments for depression, either because they hope to avoid drug-related side effects or because they are reluctant to see a doctor for their depression. Such self-treatment can put people at risk, however. For one thing, a person who self-medicates may not realize the depth of his or her depression or recognize worsening symptoms. For another, herbal and other alternative remedies are not benign and have potential side effects of their own, including the risk of drug-herb interactions.

St. John's wort, an extract from a yellow flowering plant called *Hypericum perforatum*, is the best known of "natural antidepressants." The American College of Physicians and the American Society of Internal Medicine have included it in their guidelines as a short-term treatment option for mild depression, but a recently published overview of research on the herb notes that studies conducted to date have produced "inconsistent and confusing" results.

Thus, until there is clear evidence that the supplement is effective, people with major depression should avoid using St. John's wort, and those with mild-to-moderate depression should use caution and be sure to consult their doctors before using it. In addition, anyone who uses St. John's wort needs to be aware of potential side effects. Research shows that St. John's wort interferes with a range of

Fish Oil for Depression

Can an omega-3 supplement help improve your symptoms?

While many people are helped by prescription antidepressants, the idea of trying a "natural" approach to treat depression can be appealing. One option that's been gaining attention in recent years is fish oil containing omega-3 fatty acids. These supplements are already well known for their potential to protect the heart, but they're also garnering interest for their effects on the brain. Plus, they are available without a prescription and are much less expensive than antidepressants.

But does research show that fish oil can truly help relieve depression? Is it better used as an adjunct to antidepressant therapy? And is it safe to try it?

The value of omega-3s

Also known as essential fatty acids, omega-3s are a type of polyunsaturated fatty acid and are one of three kinds of naturally occurring fats in the human diet. (The others are saturated and monounsaturated fats.) Your body cannot manufacture omega-3s; they are found mainly in seafood but also in nuts, some oils and eggs, and to a small extent, red meat. Omega-3s contain large amounts of docosahexaenoic acid (DHA) and eicosapentaenoic acid (EPA), which are believed to have numerous health benefits, such as maintaining proper functioning of the nervous system.

Omega-3s are a building block of cell membranes, and it's thought that increasing omega-3 levels makes it easier for serotonin (a chemical that relays impulses between nerve cells) to pass through cell walls. Consuming more omega-3s can also increase serotonin in the body; low levels of serotonin are linked with depression. In countries with high consumption of fish and omega-3s, there tend to be low depression rates. The opposite is true, as well, as is the case in the United States.

Some experts have blamed American eating patterns for the rise in depression. As we have tried to adopt a heart-healthy diet, we have cut back on red meat and eggs—two good non-seafood sources of omega-3s. We use a lot of oils like corn, soybean and sunflower, which are low in omega-3s. And we're now eating more omega-6 fatty acids than ever before in fast food and processed foods. Historically, humans have eaten omega-3s and omega-6s in equal proportions. Now, most of us eat far more omega-6s, and the resultant rise in this type of fatty acid has paralleled the rise in depression rates. However, the increase in the depression rate is almost certainly the result of many factors, with these dietary issues as one possible contributor.

The research

Study findings on omega-3s and depression have shown inconsistent results. As with any alternative or complementary therapy, there's no standardized preparation or formula, and the Food and Drug Administration (FDA) doesn't regulate supplements the way it does prescription drugs. However, several clinical trials have shown promise.

A 2009 Canadian study examined for the first time the effectiveness of omega-3s in menopausal women with major depression as well as less severe depression. Participants who were randomized to take 1 g of omega-3 capsules a day for eight weeks reported a lessening of depression compared with a group who took a placebo, especially among those whose symptoms were less severe.

A 2010 review article of complementary therapies for depression in the *Journal of Clinical Psychiatry* found that several clinical trials have shown promising results when omega-3s are used as an adjunct to antidepressant therapy. However, the study of omega-3s' effectiveness as a stand-alone treatment for major depression has yielded limited and conflicting results. For example, a small study of 36 adults with major depression found that 2 g of DHA per day was not more effective than a placebo

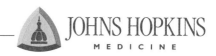

at relieving symptoms.

The type of fish oil supplement used may be a determining factor, as a study presented at the 2010 American College of Neuropsychopharmacology Conference showed. Researchers conducted a meta-analysis of 15 randomized, placebo-controlled studies on the use of omega-3s to treat depression. They found that DHA, when used alone, did not significantly improve depressive symptoms compared with a placebo. But supplements composed of EPA or a combination of DHA and EPA (with EPA predominant) were consistently effective.

Should you take omega-3s?

While this research is encouraging, larger studies need to be done to confirm the effectiveness of omega-3s for different types of depression and to determine proper dosages. While the study on fish oil and depression in menopausal women found that it was more helpful for people with milder rather than severe depression, some experts have asserted that fish oil supplements—like antidepressants—are most helpful for severe symptoms. Fish oil supplements do not elevate mood in people who are not depressed. Fish oil also does not appear to be helpful for people with depression accompanied by an anxiety disorder. For now, it may be

potentially helpful for people with depression to take fish oil in addition to an antidepressant, but there is no evidence for using it alone or instead of traditional medications.

If you are considering adding a fish oil supplement to your treatment regimen, talk to your doctor first — and never stop taking any prescribed medication without your doctor's recommendation.

When buying a fish oil supplement, look for the United States Pharmacopeia (USP) seal on the packaging. Although it doesn't make any claims about the effectiveness of a product, this labeling ensures that the product meets safety, purity and consistency standards. Based on the research discussed above, you may also want to look for formulations that contain more EPA than DHA.

The optimum dose of omega-3s for depression is not known, but the studies discussed here found improvement with dosages between 1 g and 2 g per day. As far as supplements are concerned, omega-3s are generally considered safe, and the FDA advises a dosage up to 3 g a day. Although they offer many heart-health benefits, fish oil supplements theoretically could increase the risk of bleeding if taken in high doses.

Food vs. supplements

The benefits of fish oil supplements are also present in the fish themselves. Look for oily fish such as sardines, mackerel, salmon, snapper, trout and canned white tuna, and shellfish such as mussels and oysters. Flaxseed, canola and soybean oils are also good sources of omega-3s, but only if they're unheated, as in salad dressing.

Eating these foods several times a week could provide enough omega-3 fatty acids to ease depression—provided you like fish or aren't a strict vegetarian. Many people are concerned about mercury consumption from eating fish. Farm-raised salmon, for example, can be an alternative because it doesn't contain mercury, but depending on what these fish are fed, they may not contain enough omega-3s.

Although there are certainly dietary sources of omega-3s, supplements may be the easiest, safest and most convenient way for many people to get an adequate amount of omega-3 fatty acids. Side effects are minor and include burping or an unpleasant taste. Just be wary of cod liver oil. While it is a good source of omega-3s, it contains too much vitamin A to be safe in large doses. ∎

medications, including those prescribed to treat depression, heart disease, seizures and some cancers. The supplement may also cause increased sensitivity to the sun.

Another supplement widely touted for treating depression is S-adenosylmethionine (also called SAM-e, pronounced "sammy"). But results of the published studies that purport to show the benefits of SAM-e are not at all convincing, and there are troubling hints that it may trigger mania in susceptible people.

Researchers have studied melatonin for SAD, but there is limited information on the optimal dose and timing. In addition, melatonin is a hormone and thus should be taken only with your doctor's knowledge.

Treatment of Bipolar Disorder with Medications

The goal of treating bipolar disorder is to prevent and control manic and depressive episodes, thereby creating a stable mood. (For more information on the drugs used to treat bipolar disorder, see the chart on pages 38-41.)

The core treatment is mood-stabilizing medication. Lithium was the first medication to be approved for treating mania, and it remains the mainstay of treatment today. Blood levels of lithium are measured regularly to ensure adequate doses and avoid the dangerous effects of toxic levels. Because lithium can take more than a week to have an effect, a neuroleptic (an antipsychotic drug) or a benzodiazepine (an anti-anxiety drug) may be added to treat symptoms of acute mania. Benzodiazepines should be used with caution, however, because of the risk of dependency and abuse. They can also disinhibit some manic patients, escalating inappropriate behavior.

Instead of lithium, doctors may choose to use other mood-stabilizing medications—carbamazepine (Equetro), valproic acid (Depakene, Depakote) or lamotrigine (Lamictal)—in combination with one another or with neuroleptics or benzodiazepines to treat acute mania. The neuroleptic drugs aripiprazole (Abilify), olanzapine (Zyprexa), quetiapine (Seroquel), risperidone (Risperdal) and ziprasidone (Geodon) have also been approved for treating manic episodes. Valproic acid and neuroleptics are also good options for people who have what's known as mixed states—simultaneous symptoms of mania and depression.

A neuroleptic drug is prescribed in combination with a mood-stabilizing drug when manic episodes are severe or involve hallucinations or delusional ideas. Neuroleptics are usually taken only for short periods because of their neurological side effects, which include

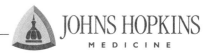

repetitive, involuntary, purposeless movements or twitches (known as tardive dyskinesia or tardive dystonia) that may not go away even if medication is stopped. These side effects occur less often with some newer (or atypical) neuroleptics, such as Zyprexa and Risperdal. These drugs are also linked with a condition called neuroleptic malignant syndrome, which includes symptoms such as muscle stiffness or spasms, high fever, and confusion or disorientation.

A new episode of mild or moderate depression in people with bipolar disorder is typically treated with a mood stabilizer such as lithium. If the depression is severe, only then would an antidepressant drug be added to the mood stabilizer. (Lithium has been shown to be effective in preventing suicide, and antidepressants must be used with caution in people with bipolar disorder.) If the depression involves psychotic symptoms, the person may need to take neuroleptic medication in addition to the mood stabilizer and antidepressant.

The reason antidepressants must be used with extreme care in people with bipolar disorder is that they can stimulate a manic episode or cause rapid cycling between depression and mania. This is particularly true for tricyclic antidepressants. Despite the presumed risk and lack of proven benefit, it's estimated that 50 to 70 percent of people with bipolar disorder are prescribed antidepressants. Each individual's situation must be assessed, since some clinical situations—such as anxiety—may be the reason for including an antidepressant in the treatment.

SSRIs and other relatively new antidepressants, such as Wellbutrin or Effexor, are the most likely drugs to be used. In addition, Symbyax—a combination of an atypical neuroleptic (olanzapine) and an SSRI (fluoxetine)—has been approved by the FDA to treat depressive episodes in people with bipolar disorder.

Despite the risk of mania, according to a study in the *American Journal of Psychiatry*, people with bipolar disorder whose depression responded to treatment with antidepressant medication (in addition to their other medications) had a low incidence of relapse into depression or mania during the first year after the depression eased if they remained on antidepressant medication during that time.

Long-term treatment of bipolar disorder

People who have had at least two episodes in five years (that is, at least two manic episodes, two depressive episodes, or one manic and one depressive episode) or three serious lifetime episodes will need to take medication over the long term, even when they experience no symptoms. This can be difficult for people to accept

Drugs for the Treatment of Bipolar Disorder 2012*

Drug type: Brand (generic)	Typical daily dosage[†]	How they appear to work
Mood stabilizers		
Depakene (valproic acid[‡])[§][‖]	250-2,000 mg	Mechanism of action is unknown.
Depakote (divalproex[‡])[§] [‖]	250-2,000 mg	
Lithobid (lithium[‡])[§]	600-1,800 mg	
Anticonvulsants		
Equetro (carbamazepine[‡])	400-1,600 mg	Suppress excessive and abnormal firing of neurons, but their exact mechanism in treating bipolar disorder is not established.
Lamictal (lamotrigine[‡])[§]	200-400 mg	
Lamictal ODT (orally disintegrating tablets)	200-400 mg	
Neurontin (gabapentin[‡])	300-1,800 mg	
Topamax (topiramate[‡])	200-1,000 mg	
Trileptal (oxcarbazepine[‡])	1,200 mg	
Atypical neuroleptics		
Abilify (aripiprazole)	15-30 mg	Symptoms of bipolar disorder may be produced by overactivity of dopamine. By blocking dopamine receptors, neuroleptics may reduce the activity of dopamine, producing antipsychotic and tranquilizing effects by preventing overstimulation of nerve cells.
Clozaril, FazaClo ODT (clozapine[‡])	12.5-450 mg	
Geodon (ziprasidone)[§]	40-160 mg	
Risperdal (risperidone)[§]	2-6 mg	
Risperdal Consta (long-acting injection)	25-50 mg every 2 weeks	
Seroquel (quetiapine)[§]	100-800 mg	
Zyprexa (olanzapine)[§]	5-20 mg	
Neuroleptics (typical)[¶]		
Permitil, Prolixin (fluphenazine[‡])	2.5-20 mg	Produce antipsychotic and tranquilizing effects by blocking dopamine receptors and preventing overstimulation of nerve cells.
Haldol (haloperidol[‡])	2-20 mg	
Atypical neuroleptic/selective serotonin reuptake inhibitor		
Symbyax (olanzapine/fluoxetine)[§]	3/25-12/50 mg	Increases the availability of the neurotransmitters serotonin, norepinephrine and dopamine to treat depression associated with bipolar disorder.

See chart legend on pages 40-41.

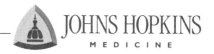

Common side effects

Depakene and Depakote can cause drowsiness, dizziness, nausea and other gastrointestinal symptoms, appetite loss, weight gain or loss, transient hair loss, hand tremor. They have also been linked with severe cases of pancreatitis (symptoms include abdominal pain, nausea, vomiting and/or anorexia). Both may also cause liver failure; symptoms include malaise, weakness, lethargy, swelling and vomiting. Regular liver function tests will be necessary.

Lithium may cause gastrointestinal discomfort, nausea, vertigo, muscle weakness, a dazed feeling, tremor, fatigue, thirst.

Equetro may cause drowsiness, weakness, blurred or double vision, dizziness, unsteadiness, nausea, sun sensitivity.

Dizziness, fatigue, poor coordination, altered vision, nausea, vomiting, headache, difficulty concentrating, impaired memory, sleepiness, insomnia. Lamictal may cause serious rashes, especially when used with Depakene without dosage adjustment, requiring hospitalization and termination of treatment.

Drowsiness, headache, dizziness, constipation, weight gain or loss, nausea, abdominal pain, tremor or twitches, muscle cramps, restlessness, salivation, dry mouth. Atypical neuroleptics increase the risk of death in elderly patients with dementia. Clozaril and FazaClo ODT have more potential side effects than other drugs in this class. They may increase the risk of elevated blood glucose and diabetes. They also can put you at risk for serious illnesses such as agranulocytosis (a decrease in the number of white blood cells that increases the risk of infected lesions of the throat and gastrointestinal tract) and myocarditis (inflammation of the walls of the heart), seizures and low blood pressure. See a doctor immediately if you experience signs of neuroleptic malignant syndrome (characterized by muscle stiffness or spasms, high fever, and confusion or disorientation) or infection (fever, chills, sweating and fatigue).

Blurred vision, stiffness, drowsiness, tremor, dry mouth, decreased sweating, sensitivity to cold and sun, persistent restlessness, loss of coordination, involuntary twitches and muscle spasms (risk highest in elderly women taking high doses). Patients taking neuroleptics experience, in rare instances, neuroleptic malignant syndrome (see atypical neuroleptic side effects).

Weight gain, sleepiness, increased appetite, weakness, swelling in legs and arms, tremors, sore throat, difficulty concentrating. Atypical neuroleptics increase the risk of death in elderly patients with dementia. See a doctor immediately if you experience signs of neuroleptic malignant syndrome (characterized by muscle stiffness or spasms, high fever, and confusion or disorientation) or infection (fever, chills, sweating and fatigue).

continued on the next page

Drugs for the Treatment of Bipolar Disorder 2012* (continued)

Drug type: Brand (generic)	Typical daily dosage†	How they appear to work
Antidepressants		
All types of antidepressants can be used (with caution) to treat depression in people with bipolar disorder. See the chart on pages 24-27 for more information on these medications.		
Benzodiazepines#		
Ativan (lorazepam‡)	2-6 mg	Increase activity of gamma-aminobutyric acid (GABA), a neurotransmitter that inhibits the excessive firing of certain neurons.
Klonopin (clonazepam‡)	0.5-4 mg	

* This list represents the most commonly prescribed drugs for bipolar disorder. Depressive episodes in bipolar disorder are often treated with a combination of mood stabilizers and antidepressant medications. Manic episodes are often treated with a combination of mood stabilizers and neuroleptic medications (either typical or atypical). Anticonvulsants are potential mood stabilizers. Benzodiazepines are often used to treat agitation and related symptoms.

† These dosages represent an average range for the treatment of bipolar disorder and may differ from the dosage prescribed by your doctor. The precise effective dosage varies from person to person and depends on many factors. Do not make any change to your medication without consulting your doctor. *Starting dosages tend to be lower for older patients.*

once they stabilize and begin to feel well again. However, research clearly shows that bipolar disorder is a chronic, cyclic disease and that the consequences of going off medication can be tragic. Treatment usually involves a mood stabilizer; other medications may be added on a short-term basis if depression or mania worsens or if symptoms such as impulsivity, irritability or poor concentration develop. A person on long-term treatment for bipolar disorder will need periodic blood tests to monitor blood levels of the medication and to check for any serious side effects, such as liver, kidney or thyroid problems.

Sleeping problems are common in people with bipolar disorder because mania can cause a reduced need for sleep and depression can cause insomnia. Benzodiazepines and certain neuroleptics may help promote sleep but are given only for short periods.

Sometimes a depressive episode occurs in someone who has been doing well with long-term treatment (known as breakthrough depression). When this happens, there are a number of treatment options. Those who experience mild-to-moderate depression may be given a higher dosage of their mood stabilizer. (In some instances, however, the mood stabilizer may actually induce mild depression, and the doctor may choose to lower the drug dosage.) If depression is severe, the person may be given an

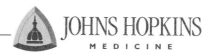

Common side effects

Dizziness, loss of coordination, drowsiness, lightheadedness, slurred speech, unsteady gait. See a doctor immediately if you experience symptoms of infection (fever, chills, sweating and fatigue) or problems with behavior (anger, depression, hallucinations or difficulty concentrating) or memory.

‡ Generic version available at lower cost.

§ Lithium, Depakene, Depakote, Lamictal, Symbyax, Zyprexa, Seroquel, Risperdal and Geodon are the only drugs approved by the Food and Drug Administration (FDA) for the treatment of bipolar disorder. Although the remaining drugs in this chart do not have FDA approval for treating bipolar disorder specifically, they are nonetheless commonly prescribed for this use.

‖ Depakene and Depakote are anticonvulsants as well as mood stabilizers.

¶ These are the highest-potency neuroleptics. Many other neuroleptics can be used to treat bipolar disorder.

Many benzodiazepines can be used to treat people with bipolar disorder. Lorazepam (Ativan) and clonazepam (Klonopin) are the most frequently used. See the chart on pages 60-61 for a more complete list of benzodiazepines.

SSRI or a second mood stabilizer. Rapid cycling between mania and depression despite long-term treatment precludes use of antidepressants.

Psychotherapy

Most people think of psychotherapy simply as counseling. In fact, the term *psychotherapy* is used to describe a variety of talk therapies that treat emotional, behavioral, personality and psychiatric disorders. It involves a commitment to a series of appointments with a licensed mental health professional, enabling a relationship to form between the therapist and the individual. This relationship focuses on helping the person cope with or avoid factors contributing to his or her condition, with the overall goals being personal development and self-understanding. Like any medical treatment, it has advantages and disadvantages.

Psychotherapy is commonly used to treat people with depression. It has proven effective in treating mild and moderate forms and can be combined with drug therapy to treat all degrees of depression.

Advantages

A major advantage over treatment with medication is that psychotherapy has few physiological side effects—an especially important consideration for older adults who are often taking more than one type of medication. In addition, it offers the possibility of effective treatment for those who have not responded to medications.

Disadvantages

A disadvantage is that psychotherapy typically takes longer than drug therapy to produce benefits that are noticeable to the person receiving treatment—six to eight weeks or longer for psychotherapy, compared with four to six weeks for medication. Also, psychotherapy alone is not effective in people with severe depression or bipolar disorder.

Depending on the severity of the depression and other factors specific to each individual, a therapist selects a combination of techniques from the range of psychotherapeutic approaches. Regardless of the particular approach, the essential foundation of all psychotherapy is the establishment of a trusting relationship with the therapist. This allows the patient to share confidences, life experiences, and problems. If psychotherapy alone leads to no improvement by six weeks, or if a person has only a partial or weak response by 12 weeks, medication should be strongly considered.

Although people with bipolar disorder should be on medication, they can also benefit from psychotherapy. Environmental factors such as stress may trigger episodes of mania or depression, and counseling can help a person identify and deal with these triggers. It can also help the person gain insight into his or her condition, confront the dysfunctional thinking often associated with bipolar disorder, and improve his or her ability to handle work, family and financial challenges. Furthermore, counseling that involves the individual's family can help educate relatives about the disorder. A recent study found that people with bipolar disorder who combined psychotherapy and medication had a 94 percent recovery rate in an average time of 113 days, compared with 52 percent of those who took medication and had only a brief psychoeducational intervention.

Unfortunately, a person who is in an acute manic state would likely be unable to attend or benefit from therapy. For those with mania or severe depression who do not respond to drug treatments or psychotherapy, electroconvulsive therapy may be needed (see "ECT: Effective Treatment for Severe Depression" on pages 48-49).

Interpersonal therapy

Also known as crisis intervention, interpersonal therapy is most effective when depression results from a major life event, such as the death of a spouse, the loss of a job, divorce or another difficult life transition. Because the depressive symptoms stem from an immediate problem, the goal is to help the person cope with the stressor by improving self-awareness, resolving emotional conflicts and possibly making some behavioral changes. Interpersonal therapy can be extremely effective at helping individuals restore balance to their lives.

Psychodynamic therapy

This form of psychotherapy focuses on an individual's past experiences in an attempt to understand present-day conflicts and feelings about recent life changes, such as retirement or grief. This therapy attempts to treat the "whole person" rather than just the symptoms of depression. A crucial component of the therapy is transference—the transfer of feelings about important childhood figures from the patient onto the therapist, who then works to help the patient resolve residual past conflicts. This therapy can be effective in helping a person overcome destructive personality patterns.

Supportive therapy

Supportive therapy teaches individuals about their illness, with the idea that a better understanding of the mood disorder will enable the person to set more realistic and tangible goals. In supportive therapy, the person is encouraged to focus on current challenges and relationships and develop strategies for dealing with them. The therapy is goal oriented, and the individual works with the therapist to set goals. The person's family members or close friends may be included in counseling or education sessions.

Behavioral therapy

This type of therapy is based on the premise that depressed people have learned destructive patterns of thinking and acting, and these patterns cause and/or prolong their depression. Counseling is provided to improve social skills, problem solving and self-control and to change how a person reacts to problems. Behavioral therapy emphasizes step-by-step improvements in behavior and is most often effective when the problem is clearly defined. Although less studied in the treatment of depression, behavioral therapy has been useful in relieving some types of anxiety states, such as obsessive-compulsive disorder and phobias.

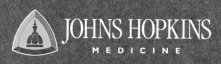
JOHNS HOPKINS
MEDICINE

The Power of Prayer

Can religious beliefs or spirituality help your mood disorder?

Medication and psychotherapy can be effective treatments for depression and anxiety, but many people also turn to a higher power for help. Prayer can be very comforting during times of grief and pain. For example, a *New England Journal of Medicine* study reported that 90 percent of Americans turned to religion following the events of September 11, 2001, to help them cope with their distress.

While some research has suggested that religion may contribute to or worsen mental illnesses, more studies suggest that religion and spirituality appear to do more good than harm.

Background
At first glance, religion and medicine seem to be at odds, but this split is relatively recent. In the United States, the first mental hospitals were run by priests in local monasteries. Religion was thought to be a civilizing influence on patients, who were allowed to attend religious services as a reward for good behavior. But in the late 19th century, mental health pioneers Jean Charcot and Sigmund Freud began to link religion with hysteria and neuroses,

and mental health treatment lost its religious component.

Today, psychiatrists are increasingly willing to incorporate religion into their practice upon the request of their patients. In fact, psychiatry as a discipline is starting to recognize the potential benefits of religion in their patients' treatment. For example, the American College of Graduate Medical Education requires that programs provide training in religious or spiritual factors that influence psychological development.

Religion and depression
A 2009 review article from Duke University examined research on the relationships between religion and depression, suicide, anxiety, psychotic disorders and substance abuse. Out of 724 published studies, more than half found that religious beliefs had a statistically significant positive impact on mental health. Among 93 observational studies, two-thirds found that more-religious people had significantly lower rates of depression or fewer depressive symptoms. And among eight randomized clinical trials, people who participated

in religious-based psychological interventions had faster symptom improvement than those in secular-based therapy or a control group.

Religious beliefs may be especially helpful for people with medical conditions who suffer from depression. The review article highlights a study of 1,000 people with depression who also suffered from congestive heart failure or chronic obstructive pulmonary disease. Those who were the most religious recovered from their depression 50 percent faster than other patients.

Caregivers may also benefit from having spiritual beliefs—one study found that religious caregivers of recently deceased cancer patients were significantly less likely to develop major depression 13 months later. Similar results were found in other studies for caregivers of people with Alzheimer's disease.

Religion and anxiety
For many people, turning to religion and prayer during stressful times seems natural and even somewhat universal. The expression "there are no atheists in

Cognitive therapy
The aim of cognitive therapy is to reverse a person's destructive and exaggerated belief that his or her weaknesses and inadequacies doom him or her to future failure. The therapist not only encourages the individual to recognize that these views are distorted—by listing positive attributes or past and present successes, for example—but also attempts to bolster confidence by demonstrating that the person can successfully complete increasingly challenging "assignments."

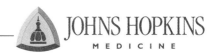

JOHNS HOPKINS
MEDICINE

foxholes" is well known. According to the Duke review article, these coping mechanisms can be helpful in reducing anxiety. Out of seven randomized clinical trials, six found that religious people who received religious interventions for generalized anxiety disorder reduced their anxiety more quickly than religious people who received secular or standard treatment.

The review also highlighted one clinical trial in which 56 people with panic disorder were treated with group cognitive-behavioral therapy. Participants who said religion was very important to them had significantly better symptom improvement and lower perceived stress 12 months later.

However, religious beliefs that focus on guilt and sin can actually increase anxiety. In a study of 100 women with gynecological cancer, those who said they felt that God was punishing them, had deserted them or was unable to make a difference had significantly higher anxiety than those who did not.

Why it may help
As with many alternative therapies, the ways in which spirituality may help—or hinder—recovery from depression and anxiety aren't fully understood. Some of the benefit may be social. For example, people who attend religious services regularly and are part of a community may receive valuable support. Attendance at religious services is also associated with other healthy behaviors such as seeking out preventive health care, engaging in physical activity and avoiding risky behaviors—all of which may improve mental health.

Can spirituality help you?
If you're a member of a faith community, you may find that speaking with your clergyperson or becoming more involved with services and activities may be helpful. If you don't have a religious background, anything that helps you feel centered and connected, such as simple prayers, meditation or mindfulness—a state of active, open attention on the present often used as a stress management tool—may be helpful. Here are some suggestions on how to incorporate spirituality into your life:

• **Bring up your faith or spirituality to your mental health professional.** He or she may not ask about it, but your religious or spiritual background is an important part of who you are and how your mind works.

• **Give prayer a try.** Some people are able to pray spontaneously, while others would rather read something already written. If you would feel more comfortable with a set prayer, look for a book or ask your clergyperson for suggestions.

• **Find a prayer group.** Ask your religious organization if it has a prayer support group for people with mental health issues or if they know of one nearby.

• **Go online.** The National Alliance on Mental Illness has an outreach program to those who want to approach mental illness from a faith perspective. NAMI's FaithNet (nami.org/namifaithnet) has articles, resources and an online discussion group.

• **Learn to meditate.** Evidence suggests that meditation may help with depression and anxiety. Meditation can be as simple as repeating a mantra—a calming word or phrase—while focusing on your breathing. ■

The treatment generally requires a series of sessions over several months. It is often combined with behavioral therapy, known as cognitive-behavioral therapy (CBT).

A recent review of 25 studies found that people undergoing CBT for generalized anxiety disorder were significantly more likely to have reduced anxiety at the end of treatment than those receiving no treatment.

Psychoanalytic therapy

The psychoanalytic theory of depression derives from the Freudian concept that altered mood develops because of anger directed toward oneself. The theory asserts that curing depression requires exposing the cause of the anger and confronting it in a constructive and realistic manner. The patient meets with the therapist three to five times a week in a stream-of-consciousness, free-associative atmosphere that involves minimal feedback from the therapist. Because classic psychoanalysis requires years of treatment, it is not suitable for managing acute depression. It is used infrequently in its classic form today, although aspects of the Freudian approach have survived under psychodynamic therapy.

Group therapy

In this method, a small group of people with similar problems meet regularly to discuss their troubles under the guidance of a therapist. Participants can share personal feelings, experiences and solutions in a supportive atmosphere. The resulting interaction often reduces feelings of isolation and can heighten awareness and understanding of personal problems. It is useful for people who benefit from feedback from peers.

Finding a therapist

If you think you have depression or bipolar disorder, you do not necessarily have to see a psychiatrist. Many people with mood disorders are treated by their primary care physician, who can identify other medical conditions that could be responsible for the symptoms. If the diagnosis does turn out to be a mood disorder, your primary care physician can initiate drug therapy, coordinate care from other specialists or both.

Many kinds of mental health professionals are available—psychiatrists, psychologists, psychiatric nurses and social workers. Which therapist is best for you? That depends on several factors, including how severe your symptoms are and the cost of treatment. No matter what type of therapy you select, keep in mind that it may take some time and research to find the right therapist. A family physician will be able to provide some recommendations, but other resources are available as well. Local medical societies, university medical centers, and national mental health organizations may be able to provide assistance. Also check community mental health clinics, local schools, and religious organizations, which sometimes offer inexpensive or even free counseling programs.

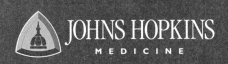

Compatibility is extremely important, and it may take more than one referral to find a comfortable counseling relationship. It is also important to ask about a therapist's education and professional licenses, either before making an appointment or during the first visit. You can get a sense of a therapist by describing your condition and asking the therapist how he or she would treat it. Reputable practitioners will not object to requests for information about their background and will understand your desire to interview other therapists.

Electroconvulsive Therapy

Many people think electroconvulsive therapy (ECT) is a thing of the past, but it is still being used today, given its effectiveness in treating major depression. In recent years, the National Institute of Mental Health, the American Psychiatric Association and the U.S. Surgeon General have all concluded that ECT is a valuable tool in the treatment of certain mental disorders, particularly depression.

Before undergoing ECT, a person with depression usually tries psychotherapy, antidepressant medication or a combination of the two. While these treatments are often effective, they take time to work. This delay can be dangerous for people whose depression is accompanied by intense suicidal thoughts or delusions. For these individuals, ECT can work much more quickly than antidepressants and is therefore a good option (see "ECT: Effective Treatment for Severe Depression" on pages 48-49).

ECT can help other people as well. It may be recommended when antidepressant medications do not work. It can also be useful for older people who cannot tolerate antidepressants and for pregnant women if there is concern that medication might affect the health of the fetus. People suffering from bipolar disorder or schizophrenia may also benefit from ECT.

No one is sure how ECT helps certain mental disorders. It may flood the brain with neurotransmitters such as serotonin and dopamine, which are known to play a role in conditions such as depression and schizophrenia. ECT may also help regulate hormones that play a role in these disorders.

Light Therapy

Some people with seasonal affective disorder (SAD) can be successfully treated with exposure to bright light. In one study, 57 percent of 191 people with SAD responded to light therapy. In another study, light therapy was comparable in effectiveness to antidepressant therapy but worked faster and caused fewer side effects. And in a

LATEST RESEARCH

Looking Forward Helps Patients with Depression

A type of therapy that teaches people how to look forward to a positive future may be helpful in treating major depression.

In a new study, researchers from Cedars-Sinai Medical Center in Los Angeles explored the possible benefits of "future-directed therapy," or FDT. According to the researchers, FDT encourages people to not dwell on the past or their current limitations, but to develop the skills that help them maintain positive expectations about the future. Skills include goal-setting, problem-solving, taking action and dealing in a constructive manner with disappointment.

In the study, 16 people with major depressive disorder chose to take 20 sessions of FDT over 10 weeks, and another 17 participated in traditional cognitive-based therapy. The people participating in FDT had significant improvements in their depression, anxiety and quality of life. They also reported that they were very satisfied with the therapy. This group had greater improvement in their depressive symptoms than the other group as measured by a standard depression questionnaire.

This was merely a pilot study, but it found evidence that this type of therapy warrants further research, including a trial in which people are randomly assigned to FDT or another type of treatment.

CNS NEUROSCIENCE & THERAPEUTICS
Published Online
March 16, 2011

ECT: Effective Treatment for Severe Depression

Electroconvulsive therapy can help when medications don't work

If you're struggling with depression and nothing seems to be working—not drugs, not talk therapy—don't lose hope. An option you may not have considered is electroconvulsive treatment (ECT), which is the most effective type of antidepressant treatment available. ECT can be a lifeline for people with depression that's life-threatening or difficult to treat.

ECT used to have a bad reputation. Indeed, when it was first introduced in the late 1930s, patients would thrash around so violently that they could wind up with broken bones.

Now that patients receive anesthesia and a muscle relaxant, the treatment is virtually painless and seizures are barely visible. It's even safe enough to be used in pregnant women and people with heart disease. Each year, an estimated 100,000 people in the United States undergo ECT for depression and other psychiatric problems. The reputation of ECT is changing dramatically.

What is ECT?
ECT involves passing a carefully controlled electrical current through a person's brain. The current needs to be strong enough to generate epileptic activity (a seizure), which is a rapid discharge of nerve impulses throughout the brain.

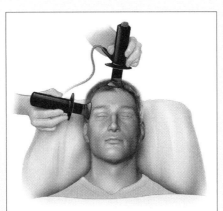

In unilateral ECT, one electrode is placed at the top of the head and the other is placed on the right temple.

After an anesthesiologist puts the patient briefly under general anesthesia and administers a muscle relaxant, a specially trained psychiatrist places two electrode pads, each about the size of a silver dollar, on two areas of the scalp. A short, controlled set of electrical pulses is then passed between the electrodes by a machine designed for this purpose. The current lasts for a couple of seconds, and the resulting epileptic discharge typically lasts for about a minute.

People wake up about five minutes after the treatment is over. Most people feel confused for the next half hour or so and may experience headache, muscle stiffness or nausea.

When it's used
In its most recent practice guidelines, the American Psychiatric Association (APA) recommends ECT as a treatment option for people with severe depression that has not responded to either drugs or psychotherapy. The APA also recommends ECT for treatment of severely depressed people who are psychotic (having hallucinations or delusions), catatonic (immobile), dangerously suicidal or starving themselves. ECT can be the best choice for people in emergency situations like these because it is so effective and tends to work more rapidly than medication.

Drugs usually take four to eight weeks to take effect, and people sometimes try two, three or even four medications in an effort to find one that works for them. The process can take months. By contrast, ECT usually takes just two or three weeks to work. Sometimes, improvement is seen after just one treatment. Most people who undergo ECT will require treatment two or three times a week, for a total of six to 12 sessions.

Benefits and risks
Multiple clinical trials have shown ECT to be effective for depression. In the Consortium for Research in ECT (CORE) study of nearly 400 people, 86 percent of people who had ECT saw their depression go away. This is sig-

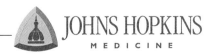

nificantly higher than the 21 to 30 percent remission rate with a single medication trial.

Despite its effectiveness, treatment with ECT is far from trivial. Like any epileptic activity, ECT can interfere with memory. It's common to have trouble learning new information in the weeks after ECT treatments, although this effect is temporary. Some people also forget events that occurred immediately before the sessions.

Even more disturbing is the small percentage of people who complain of persistent memory problems—a phenomenon for which few data exist. Many people who have ECT are older and already experiencing memory loss, so it's difficult to know whether the treatment is at fault. In fact, ECT often improves memory because depression itself often impairs cognitive function.

Reducing the side effects

Doctors have been working to refine ECT in an effort to minimize side effects such as confusion and memory loss. Two of these refinements are unilateral ECT and the use of ultra-brief pulses.

At Johns Hopkins, doctors generally use unilateral ECT instead of bilateral ECT. In unilateral ECT, one electrode is placed at the top of the head and the other is placed on the right temple so the current passes through only the right side of the brain. In bilateral ECT, one electrode is placed on the left side of the head and the other is placed on the right side so the current passes through both sides of the brain.

Hopkins also regularly employs narrower electrical pulses known as ultra-brief pulses, especially for people receiving ECT as outpatients. These narrower pulses last less than half a millisecond, whereas traditional pulses last for 1 millisecond. Researchers have found that ultra-brief pulses work well and are associated with less memory loss than traditional pulses, although it may take patients a few more treatments to recover than with treatment using traditional pulses.

Keeping depression at bay

An important shortcoming of ECT is that its effects often wear off after just a few weeks. Most people take antidepressants after ECT to keep depression at bay, an approach that tends to work even in those whose depression didn't respond to drugs initially.

People who aren't able to take medication—or whose depression comes back despite antidepressant treatment—have the option of maintenance ECT. This may involve a treatment every two to four weeks.

Other potential treatments for depression that doesn't respond to drugs or talk therapy include transcranial magnetic stimulation, vagus nerve stimulation and light therapy. None of these appear to be nearly as effective as ECT, however.

A lifesaving treatment

Although ECT is considered relatively safe, an estimated 1 in 10,000 patients die due to the procedure. This rate is about the same as that associated with minor surgery with similar anesthesia. There is also a theoretical risk of heart problems and injuries such as broken bones, although modern techniques and careful monitoring have made these highly unlikely.

Those who treat depression emphasize that it's important to put the risks of ECT in context. Although far from perfect, ECT is sometimes the only thing that works to relieve the intense suffering of depression. Because as many as 15 percent of people with depression die due to the disorder, mainly by suicide, ECT can be a lifesaver. For people with severe depression, who are often completely unable to function in their daily activities—unable to eat or take care of themselves—ECT can lead to remarkable recoveries. ■

major review of 173 published studies, bright-light therapy yielded substantial relief for both SAD and mild-to-moderate depression that was not linked to seasonal changes.

Light therapy involves sitting in front of a bank of full-spectrum fluorescent lights for 30 to 60 minutes each day. Improvement can often be seen within a few days, with symptoms disappearing after two to three weeks. Continued light therapy is needed to prevent a relapse. Although commercially available light boxes are advertised for depressed people, these devices are not approved by the FDA. Light therapy should be used only with your doctor's guidance, as it can cause side effects when used improperly. For instance, light therapy may trigger manic symptoms in people who have bipolar disorder.

Supplemental Treatments

Other healthy behaviors that can improve recovery success rates include regular exercise, improved sleep and good nutrition.

Exercise

Numerous studies have shown that exercise can alleviate depression and improve mood. One review of 14 studies found that aerobic exercise three times a week for at least five weeks was more effective than a placebo at relieving symptoms of mild-to-moderate depression and was just as effective as psychotherapy. The benefits of aerobic exercise in these studies lasted up to a year, especially among those who continued exercising. Exercise was also shown to be more cost effective than other treatments.

No one is sure exactly how exercise relieves depression. An increase in aerobic fitness may play a role but cannot be entirely responsible because nonaerobic exercise, such as weight training, can have similar effects. Some researchers have theorized that exercise, like most antidepressant medications, increases the activity of serotonin and/or norepinephrine. Exercise also stimulates the release of endorphins, which are hormones that reduce pain and can induce euphoria. Exercise may provide an outlet for pent-up anger and frustration as well. In addition, it may improve disturbed sleep, which can be a symptom of and an aggravating factor in depression. Finally, there are some reports that even brief exposure to natural daylight— as with a walk outside during the middle of the day or other outdoor exercise—helps people with SAD.

Some of the effects of exercise may have more to do with psychology than physiology. For instance, exercise may give people a sense of self-mastery or control over their depression or anxiety, which can lead to a reduction in symptoms.

To increase your level of physical activity, begin by making small changes in your daily life. Try parking your car farther away from the store or mall to increase the amount of time you spend walking. When possible, take the stairs instead of an elevator. Also, try to decrease the amount of time you spend in sedentary activities, such as watching television. Your goal should be at least 30 minutes of moderately intense activity, such as swimming, bicycling, gardening, raking leaves or brisk walking on most days of the week. However, any increase in activity can be beneficial.

Sleep

Most people experience mild irritability or mood changes when they have insomnia, but sleep deprivation can have an even greater impact on those with mood disorders. Chronic sleep deprivation and irregular sleep habits not only worsen depression but may also interfere with its treatment. Sleep disturbances can even trigger a manic episode in some people. Focusing on getting regular, adequate sleep is a crucial part of controlling symptoms and increasing the benefits of other mood disorder treatments. (In some depressed people, though, controlled sleep deprivation may result in very brief, temporary improvements in depressive symptoms.)

Nutrition

If you suffer from depression, one of the most important things you can do to help yourself is avoid alcohol. There is no question that alcohol exacerbates depression. It is, after all, a chemical depressant.

As for general nutrition, some individuals with mild depression or dysthymia report that they feel better when they eat more foods containing omega-3 fatty acids (such as salmon and other fatty fish) or complex carbohydrates (such as beans and whole grains). However, the interplay between food and mood is not well understood.

Malnutrition, particularly folic acid and vitamin B_{12} deficiencies, has been associated with depression in older people. Eating a well-balanced diet will help provide the full range of nutrients your body needs to stay healthy in general.

Future Treatments

For individuals whose depression is not alleviated by standard therapies, new treatment options are under investigation. At the forefront

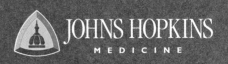

LATEST RESEARCH

Light May Help Treat Major Depression

Exposure to bright light may help lighten the symptoms of major depression.

In a new study, Dutch researchers included 89 people with major depressive disorder (MDD) who were ages 60 and older. The participants were randomly assigned to get an hour of exposure every morning for three weeks to either bright-light treatment or a dim red light, which was used as a placebo.

The researchers measured the subjects' depression at the beginning of the study, after three weeks of treatment and three weeks after the end of the treatment. The bright-light group had a 7 percent better improvement in depression scores at the end of the treatment compared with the placebo group. Three weeks after the end of treatment, symptoms kept improving in the bright-light group but not the placebo group.

In addition, at the end of treatment the bright-light group had a better improvement in sleep efficiency (the amount of time they spent actually sleeping after they fell asleep) than the other group, and they got out of bed faster after they woke up.

Bright-light treatment may be an important supplemental treatment for people who do not fully respond to antidepressant treatment.

ARCHIVES OF GENERAL PSYCHIATRY
Volume 68, page 61
January 2011

of research are various brain-stimulating techniques, such as deep brain stimulation (DBS), which involves the implantation of a device that delivers an electrical current to the brain to normalize its activity. Like the heart, the brain is an electrical organ, so stimulating it with a small electrical current is an efficient way to precisely target areas that are malfunctioning—more efficiently than drug therapy, in fact, which tends to affect the whole brain and often causes side effects. Although results of small trials have been encouraging, the finer points of the procedure are still being debated—the precise areas of the brain to stimulate, the optimal number of electrodes to implant and the voltages to use. DBS is not without risk. It is, after all, brain surgery, which carries with it the chance of hemorrhage (excessive bleeding) in the brain, infection and even death. The DBS device can malfunction, and the batteries typically need to be replaced after four to five years. In addition, doctors need to carefully monitor the multiple medications patients are typically taking to ensure that drug side effects and interactions are minimized.

Besides DBS, studies have shown that vagus nerve stimulation (VNS) may help people with treatment-resistant depression. A vagus nerve stimulator is a small, surgically implanted device designed to stimulate the brain periodically through the vagus nerve—a major nerve that passes from the brain through the neck and chest into the abdomen.

Another treatment method under investigation is rapid transcranial magnetic stimulation (rTMS). In this technique, an electromagnetic coil is placed on the scalp (but not implanted). A high-intensity current passes through the coil and produces a powerful magnetic field that affects the function of the underlying brain cells. Some studies have shown that rTMS performed in the frontal areas of the brain can have antidepressant effects. A 2010 study found that 14 percent of participants saw improvements in their depressive symptoms after rTMS compared with 5 percent of a control group.

Additional drugs are also being tested for treating depression. These include drugs that stimulate the production of gamma-aminobutyric acid (GABA, a neurotransmitter that suppresses the action of nerve cells); medications that block the action of glutamate (a neurotransmitter that stimulates nerve cells); drugs that block substance P (a protein originally investigated for its role in pain); and blockers of corticotropin-releasing factor receptors, which play a role in the body's reaction to stress.

Even the wrinkle fighter botulinum toxin (Botox) is under

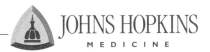

investigation. In one small preliminary trial of 10 women, it was injected into facial muscles to discourage frowning, resulting in a reduction in depressive symptoms.

ANXIETY DISORDERS

Anxiety is a common, normal and often useful response to life's challenges and dangers. But in people who suffer from an anxiety disorder, anxiety levels spin out of control, causing psychological and physical symptoms that interfere with normal functioning, appear even in the absence of obvious external stressors, or are clearly excessive in the face of the stressors.

Researchers believe that anxiety disorders result from hyperactivity in certain areas of the brain, perhaps related to low levels of the neurotransmitter gamma-aminobutyric acid (GABA), which is responsible for keeping activity levels of nerve cells in check. Anxiety disorders also run in families.

Despite how common it is, anxiety may be undertreated: In one study, almost 20 percent of patients visiting a primary care clinic were diagnosed with at least one anxiety disorder—but 41 percent of them were receiving no treatment.

Symptoms of Anxiety

Common psychological symptoms of anxiety include irritability, intense fear, worry, difficulty concentrating and a general "keyed up" feeling. Physical symptoms include sweating, dry mouth, hot flashes or chills, dizziness, heart palpitations, muscle tension, trembling, nausea and restlessness.

Some medical conditions and drugs can cause anxiety or produce its symptoms. Alcohol withdrawal, asthma, a heart attack, an overactive thyroid and a deficiency in folate or vitamin B_{12} are examples. Drugs that might cause or mimic anxiety symptoms include bronchodilators such as ephedrine and epinephrine, psychostimulants such as methylphenidate (Ritalin) and thyroid hormone.

Effects of Anxiety on Physical Health

Some evidence suggests that chronic anxiety may lead to long-term health problems, such as hypertension (high blood pressure). An 18- to 20-year follow-up of people who participated in the Framingham

Depression and Anxiety

What to do if you suspect that you're suffering from both conditions

Depression is a common problem, affecting about one in six adults in their lifetime. You should suspect depression if you have sadness that lasts for more than two weeks and interferes with your ability to function. But what if you also feel excessively anxious? If so, you may be one of the many people who experience an anxiety disorder at the same time as depression.

A study from Harvard found that among people with depression, nearly two-thirds also had generalized anxiety disorder. The rates of co-occurring related anxiety disorders—social phobia, post-traumatic stress disorder, panic disorder, specific phobias and obsessive-compulsive disorder— in depressed people were also all greater than 40 percent.

Treating with antidepressants
Having an anxiety disorder at the same time as depression can make it harder to find a treatment that works, according to guidelines from the American Psychiatric Association, but not impossible.

Antidepressants are often effective for symptoms of both depression and anxiety. You should be aware, however, that selective serotonin reuptake inhibitors (SSRIs), such as fluoxetine (Prozac) and sertraline (Zoloft), and tricyclics, which include the drug nortriptyline (Pamelor), can make anxiety worse before making it better. For this reason, your doctor will probably start you at a low dose and slowly increase the amount you need to take.

SSRIs seem to be an especially good choice for people with social phobias or post-traumatic stress disorder. Both SSRIs and the tricyclic clomipramine (Anafranil) have been shown to help people with depression and obsessive-compulsive disorder. SSRIs are the treatment of choice for both depression and panic disorder.

Additional treatments
If an antidepressant is helping with your depression but not your anxiety, your doctor may add a benzodiazepine such as clonazepam (Klonopin) or lorazepam (Ativan)—but be aware that it's easy to become dependent on these drugs.

Also keep in mind that medication isn't the only way to treat depression and anxiety. Many people opt for psychotherapy, which can be effective for both conditions. Many studies show the greatest benefit from a combination of drugs and psychotherapy.

Although it's normal to feel sad or anxious, see your doctor if your symptoms are severe and interfere with daily functioning. ■

Heart Study found such a connection in men ages 45 to 59. None of the men had high blood pressure at the start of the study. To evaluate psychological traits that might lead to high blood pressure, participants were asked about levels of anxiety, feelings of anger and expression of anger. Men who had a high score for anxiety at the start of the study were twice as likely to develop high blood pressure than those with a low score for anxiety symptoms. Not all studies have found such an association, however.

Heart attack risk may also be increased by anxiety. A study of 30,000 men, ages 42 to 77, found that those who scored highest on a questionnaire measuring common phobias had triple the risk of a subsequent fatal heart attack than men with the lowest scores. Similar results were found in a smaller study of 1,408 men in the United

Kingdom. It is possible that the fatal heart attacks resulted from some physical consequence of phobic anxiety, such as a disturbance in the heart's rhythm or hyperventilation, which led to spasm of a coronary artery.

One large Canadian study found that among people with mental and physical health issues, anxiety was most commonly linked with lung and gastrointestinal illnesses, arthritis, allergies, thyroid problems and migraine headaches. It is possible that anxiety could trigger one or more processes—like hormonal changes—that contribute to a physical illness.

Panic Disorder

The main features of panic disorder include sudden but short-lived attacks of terror and a fear of losing control. Attacks begin without warning during nonthreatening activities. Affected individuals often go to the emergency room or consult a cardiologist because the physical symptoms are similar to those of a heart attack. (If you ever suspect that you're having a heart attack, see a doctor or go to the nearest emergency room immediately.) Panic attacks generally peak within 10 minutes and dissipate within 20 to 30 minutes. They are characterized by some combination of the following symptoms:

- Shortness of breath or hyperventilation
- Heart palpitations or a racing pulse
- Discomfort in the chest
- Dizziness, lightheadedness or feeling faint
- Choking, nausea or stomach pain
- Sweating
- Hot or cold flashes
- Trembling or shaking
- A feeling of detachment from one's surroundings or a sense of unreality
- Tingling or numbness
- Fear of dying or losing one's mind

Symptoms of depression and anxiety are common in people with panic disorder. Although both panic attacks and symptoms of depression and anxiety may improve with antidepressant medications, some people require separate medications (see "Depression and Anxiety" on page 54).

According to the National Institute of Mental Health, 6 million adults (about 3 percent of adult Americans) suffer from panic disorder each year. It is twice as common in women as in men. Attacks commonly begin in the late teens or early 20s and often

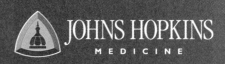

LATEST RESEARCH

Computer-Based CBT Shows Benefits

Cognitive behavioral therapy (CBT) provided via computer may be effective for treating depression and anxiety.

In a recent study, researchers combed through databases to find randomized controlled trials that compared CBT with other options in treating people with major depression, panic disorder, social phobia or generalized anxiety disorder.

Computerized CBT—given over the Internet or in a clinic—teaches the principles of cognitive behavioral therapy in a series of lessons, often with homework assignments. The advantages of computerized therapy include convenience (such as completion of the program in the evenings when there are no competing demands), ability to proceed at one's own pace to master the material, low cost and privacy.

The 22 studies the researchers gathered found that computerized CBT was superior to control situations, and the benefit was seen for all these problems. The improvements from the computerized CBT lasted for about 26 weeks of follow-up. In five studies that compared computerized CBT with face-to-face CBT, the two approaches seemed equally beneficial.

PLOS ONE
Volume 5, e13196
October 13, 2010

go undiagnosed and untreated. One study estimated that only one in four people with panic attacks receives appropriate care.

The most common complication of panic disorder is agora-phobia—fear of being in public places, especially when alone—which develops as a result of trying to avoid situations that have triggered panic attacks in the past. Left untreated, panic attacks and agoraphobia can severely restrict a person's lifestyle. Panic disorder is also associated with an increased frequency of major depression, alcohol and drug dependency, and suicide.

Generalized Anxiety Disorder

Generalized anxiety disorder (GAD) is characterized by excessive, recurrent and prolonged anxiety and worrying. People with GAD typically agonize over everyday concerns, such as job responsibilities, finances, health or family well-being or even more minor concerns as household chores, car repairs, being late for appointments or personal appearance. The focus of anxiety may shift frequently from one concern to another, and sensations may range from mild tension and nervousness to feelings of dread.

GAD affects 6.8 million adults (about 3 percent of adult Americans) each year. Although people with GAD know that the intensity, duration and frequency of their anxiety and worry are out of proportion to the actual likelihood or impact of the feared event, they still have difficulty controlling their emotions. Perpetual anxiety may impair concentration, memory and decision-making ability, decrease attention span and lead to a loss of confidence. Normal activities, such as working, socializing with friends and maintaining intimate relationships, may become difficult or even impossible.

GAD may also produce a range of physical symptoms, including heart palpitations, restlessness, sweating, headaches and nausea. Some GAD sufferers, not realizing that GAD is a treatable illness, become accustomed to their condition and assume that it is normal to feel on edge all the time. But the constant anxiety can lead to alcohol or drug abuse. The physical symptoms of GAD, along with alcohol or drug abuse, are often what finally compel a person to seek treatment.

Obsessive-Compulsive Disorder

Obsessive-compulsive disorder (OCD) is marked by recurrent, repetitive thoughts (obsessions), behaviors (compulsions) or both. People with OCD recognize that their obsessions and compulsions are unreasonable, unnecessary, intrusive and sometimes even foolish, yet they cannot resist them. Regardless of whether a person suffers from obsessions, compulsions or both, the condition interferes with day-to-day activities and relationships.

Obsessions are defined as recurring and persistent thoughts, ideas, images or impulses, sometimes of an aggressive nature, that seem to invade a person's consciousness. The sufferer will try to suppress or ignore these uncomfortable thoughts, often recognizing that they are unrealistic. Common obsessions are a fear of germs, thoughts of violent behavior (such as killing a family member), fear of making a mistake or of harming oneself or others and a constant need for reassurance.

Compulsions are ritualistic, repetitive and purposeful behaviors that are performed according to certain rules or stereotypical patterns. The behavior, although clearly excessive, temporarily relieves the tension and discomfort brought on by the obsessive thoughts. Common compulsions are rechecking to be sure doors are locked, windows are closed or an appliance is turned off; excessive neatness and organization; and repetitive hand washing that accompanies an obsession with dirt and germs.

OCD occurs in about 2.2 million adult Americans (1 percent of the adult population) and affects men and women equally. It most often starts in childhood or in the teens or early 20s. Embarrassed and upset by their behavior, most sufferers try to keep it a secret. Those with mild OCD often manage to function with only minimal interference in their daily lives. But in people with more pronounced OCD, obsessive thoughts or compulsive behaviors may be frequent or distressing enough to become incapacitating.

Probably the most common complication of the disorder is depression. Another is marked interference with social and work behaviors. Although some people with OCD experience spontaneous remission, in most the illness has an episodic course with periods of partial remission. In about 10 percent of sufferers, the course of OCD is chronic and unchanged.

Post-Traumatic Stress Disorder

Post-traumatic stress disorder (PTSD) is a form of chronic psychological stress that follows exposure to a traumatic event, such as a natural disaster, a violent crime, an accident, terrorism or warfare. The symptoms include the following:

- Recurrent, intrusive, distressing dreams and memories of the trauma
- A sudden sense that the event is recurring; experiencing flashbacks

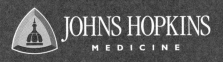
JOHNS HOPKINS
MEDICINE

LATEST RESEARCH

Deep Brain Stimulation May Help in OCD

For people with obsessive-compulsive disorder that doesn't respond to other treatments, deep brain stimulation using electrodes implanted in the brain may offer relief.

In a recent study, Dutch researchers followed 16 adults with obsessive-compulsive disorder (OCD) who had tried a variety of medications and cognitive behavioral therapy without success. The patients underwent surgery to implant the electrodes in a brain area called the nucleus accumbens. For eight months, the electrodes were stimulated, followed by a phase in which they were either turned on or off for two weeks apiece, followed by another 12 months in which they were turned on.

During the first eight-month phase, nine of the 16 patients responded to the treatment, and their scores on an obsessive-compulsive scale fell by 72 percent. During the phase when the electrodes were turned on or off, patients showed a 25 percent difference in scores between the two settings. The treatment was associated with a significant drop in depression and anxiety, but the patients noticed mild forgetfulness and trouble finding words.

More research is needed to learn which patients could benefit the most from this therapy and to discover the best place to insert the electrodes.

ARCHIVES OF GENERAL PSYCHIATRY
Volume 67, page 1061
October 2010

- Extreme distress when confronted with events that symbolize or resemble the trauma
- Attempting to avoid thoughts, feelings and activities associated with the event
- Inability to remember aspects of the trauma
- Markedly diminished interest in important activities
- Feelings of detachment and estrangement from loved ones
- Low expectations for the future
- Insomnia or excessive fatigue
- Extreme irritability
- Inability to concentrate
- Hypervigilance or an exaggerated startle response

Symptoms must last at least one month for a diagnosis of post-traumatic stress disorder. In the acute version of the syndrome, symptoms begin within six months of the trauma. The chronic syndrome may be delayed in its onset until more than six months after the event or may persist for more than six months afterward. As many as 5 percent of people involved in a major natural disaster suffer enough distress to need treatment. The numbers are closer to 28 to 34 percent for man-made traumas (such as bombings, shootings or plane crashes). Complications include anxiety, alcohol or drug abuse, depression, and family or work problems.

Overall, 7.7 million adults (3.5 percent of adult Americans) develop PTSD each year. It can develop at any age and tends to affect women more than men.

Phobic Disorders

The hallmarks of phobic disorders are persistent, irrational fears and avoidance of the specific things or activities (for example, air travel, closed spaces, certain animals or insects) that induce these fears. The diagnosis of a phobic disorder is made only when the phobia significantly impairs the individual's social functioning or work performance.

A common type of phobia is social phobia (also called social anxiety disorder), which affects 15 million adults (nearly 7 percent of the population). Social phobia is an undue fear of embarrassment in social situations. Although many people feel some anxiety when placed in a situation that forces them to meet and talk to new people, social phobia causes such an extreme reaction to this everyday aspect of life that it interferes with daily functioning (see "Overcoming Social Phobia" on pages 64-65).

Treatment of Anxiety

Treatment of anxiety does not always require medication. The use of anti-anxiety drugs depends in part on whether the person can tolerate his or her symptoms while learning to manage them. Coping measures include psychotherapy and stress-reducing therapies such as progressive muscle relaxation, biofeedback or, less commonly, yoga, self-hypnosis or meditation. In general, these approaches are designed to give people with anxiety a feeling of control over their symptoms.

If you suffer from anxiety, you can help yourself by getting adequate sleep, exercising (which aids sleep and improves self-esteem), and avoiding caffeine and alcohol. Often a person has more than one anxiety disorder; determining exactly which disorders are present can lead to better treatment. As with mood disorders, a careful evaluation by a health professional is the first step in treatment. Depending on the severity of anxiety symptoms, treatment can be managed by your primary care physician or a specialist.

General Medication Treatment

Although benzodiazepines are still commonly used to treat anxiety, two classes of antidepressant drugs—SSRIs and tricyclics—have become the first line of treatment. Serotonin and norepinephrine reuptake inhibitors and tetracyclics also are used to treat these conditions. These drugs are not habit forming and can be effective in low doses. Antidepressants are useful when a person with anxiety is also depressed (see "Depression and Anxiety" on page 54).

Tricyclics and SSRIs take several weeks to work, making them slower acting than benzodiazepines, but they do bring a fast-acting benefit to people with anxiety by promoting better sleep, which quickly improves daily functioning.

Benzodiazepines

It is thought that benzodiazepines relieve anxiety by enhancing the effects of the neurotransmitter GABA. The mechanism of action is not fully understood, however. The side effects of benzodiazepines are generally minor. They include mild disturbances of thinking and, in rare instances, slowed breathing. Two side effects of benzodiazepines, drowsiness and clumsiness, may lead to an increased risk of accidents while driving. A study from Quebec found that users of benzodiazepines had a 26 percent greater chance of having a car accident than nonusers. The increased risk for those using benzodiazepines was highest (45 percent) during the first week of therapy.

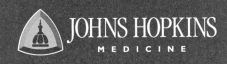

ASK THE DOCTOR

Q. *How can I best help a veteran with post-traumatic stress disorder (PTSD)?*

A. Many veterans who have returned to their families and jobs in recent years have post-traumatic stress disorder (PTSD). Some research suggests that roughly 20 percent of those who were deployed in Iraq or Afghanistan have symptoms of PTSD or depression.

Family members can help a loved one with PTSD by accompanying him or her to doctor appointments, learning how any medications or therapy are supposed to work, offering a listening ear while giving the person space as needed, organizing healthy activities such as exercise, and encouraging the person to stay socially active.

Bringing the whole family to a therapist may also be useful in helping your loved ones communicate better and giving everyone in the family tools to better deal with the PTSD. If the person with PTSD has anger issues that make communication difficult, develop a plan for how to temporarily step away from upsetting conversations when they arise and return to them later.

Employers can help someone with PTSD during working hours by allowing flexible work schedules, providing tools like checklists and reminders to help the worker stay focused and organized, and remembering that people with PTSD have some good days and some harder days.

Commonly Used Anti-anxiety Drugs 2012*

Drug type: Brand (generic)	Typical daily dosage[†]	How they appear to work
Benzodiazepines		
Ativan (lorazepam‡)	2-6 mg	Balance brain chemicals by enhancing effects of the neurotransmitter gamma-aminobutyric acid (GABA).
GenXene (clorazepate‡)	15-60 mg	
Klonopin (clonazepam‡)	0.5-4 mg	
Librium (chlordiazepoxide‡)	15-100 mg	
Niravam (alprazolam‡)	0.75-4 mg	
(oxazepam§)	30-120 mg	
Tranxene, Tranxene-SD (clorazepate‡)	15-60 mg	
Valium (diazepam‡)	4-40 mg	
Xanax (alprazolam‡)	0.75-4 mg	
Buspirone		
BuSpar (buspirone‡)	15-40 mg	Affects the actions of the neurotransmitters serotonin and dopamine in the brain.
Selective serotonin reuptake inhibitors (SSRIs)		
Celexa (citalopram‡)	20-60 mg	Block the reabsorption and inactivation of the neurotransmitter serotonin by neurons. This increases the availability of serotonin to carry messages between nerve cells.
Lexapro (escitalopram)	10-20 mg	
Luvox (fluvoxamine)	50-300 mg	
Luvox CR (fluvoxamine, controlled-release)	100-300 mg	
Paxil (paroxetine‡)	10-60 mg	
Paxil CR (paroxetine, controlled-release)	12.5-75 mg	
Prozac (fluoxetine‡)	10-60 mg	
Zoloft (sertraline‡)	25-200 mg	
Serotonin and norepinephrine reuptake inhibitors (SNRIs)		
Cymbalta (duloxetine)	40-60 mg	Block the reabsorption of serotonin and norepinephrine, increasing the availability of these neurotransmitters in the brain.
Effexor (venlafaxine‡)	75-375 mg	
Effexor XR (venlafaxine, extended-release)	75-225 mg	
(trazodone§)	150-400 mg	
Tetracyclics		
Remeron (mirtazapine‡)	15-45 mg	Block the reabsorption of serotonin and/or norepinephrine, increasing the availability of these neurotransmitters in the brain.
Remeron SolTab (mirtazapine‡)	15-45 mg	
Tricyclics		
Anafranil (clomipramine‡)	25-250 mg	Block the reabsorption of serotonin, norepinephrine and, to a lesser extent, dopamine, increasing the availability of these neurotransmitters in the brain.
Aventyl (nortriptyline‡)	75-150 mg	
Norpramin (desipramine‡)	100-300 mg	
Pamelor (nortriptyline‡)	75-150 mg	
Silenor (doxepin‡)	25-300 mg	
Tofranil (imipramine‡)	75-200 mg	

* Many of these drugs are not approved by the U.S. Food and Drug Administration (FDA) for anxiety disorders but are commonly used to treat them.

† These dosages represent an average range for the treatment of anxiety and may differ from the dosage prescribed by your doctor. The precise effective dosage varies from person to person and depends on many factors. Do not make any change to your medication without consulting your doctor. *Starting dosages tend to be lower for older patients.*

‡ Generic version available at lower cost.

§ Generic only available.

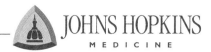

Precautions	Common side effects
Chronic use of these drugs may lead to tolerance and dependence. Antacids may decrease effectiveness. Do not drink alcohol while using.	Sedation (benzodiazepines are often purposely prescribed for their ability to induce relaxation and sleep), dizziness, weakness, unsteadiness/clumsiness, depression, headache, dry mouth, decreased sex drive, dependence.
Do not take with monoamine oxidase (MAO) inhibitors.	Dizziness, nausea, headache, nervousness, lightheadedness, excitement. Nonaddictive, less sedating than other antianxiety drugs.
Do not take with MAO inhibitors, triptans or St. John's wort. The development of a skin rash can be a sign of a serious medical problem; see a doctor immediately. If discontinuing use, reduce dosage gradually to prevent withdrawal symptoms. *Celexa only*: This drug should no longer be used at doses greater than 40 mg a day due to risk of causing abnormal changes in the electrical activity of the heart at higher doses.	Anxiety, nervousness, insomnia, drowsiness, weakness, headache, diarrhea, increased sweating, nausea, impaired sexual function, weight gain. Side effects appear to be lesser with Lexapro.
Do not take with MAO inhibitors or triptans. Effexor may increase blood pressure and/or cholesterol levels in some people; regular blood pressure and cholesterol monitoring is advised. If discontinuing use, reduce dosage gradually to prevent withdrawal symptoms.	Nausea, weakness, sweating, insomnia, drowsiness, dry mouth, dizziness, constipation, nervousness, impaired sexual function, appetite loss.
Do not take with MAO inhibitors. Caution advised with use of Remeron in the elderly because of delayed clearance of the drug, which may increase the risk of adverse effects.	Sleepiness, nausea, increased appetite, weight gain, dizziness, blurred vision, weakness, dry mouth, headache, constipation, shakiness, nervousness.
Do not take with MAO inhibitors. Do not stop treatment abruptly. It is not advisable to take tricyclic antidepressants if you have seizures, a heart disorder or glaucoma, or if you use alcohol excessively.	Dizziness on standing, drowsiness, weakness, headache, dry mouth, blurred vision, constipation, nausea, difficulty urinating, increased appetite (may include a craving for sweets), impaired sexual function, increased heart rate. Skin is more sensitive to sunlight during use of these drugs, which may result in itching, redness, discoloration of skin.

The most troublesome issues with benzodiazepine treatment are the development of tolerance (decreased effectiveness of a given dose with continued use) and both physical and psychological dependence, especially with long-term use of a drug at high doses. Physical dependence is defined by the development of a specific set of physical symptoms upon withdrawal of a drug. Psychological dependence refers to a persistent desire for the drug after it has been discontinued.

Tolerance may cause a person to request, and at times receive, increasingly larger doses to maintain benefits. In this instance, the person may be switched to an SSRI or a tricyclic drug instead of higher doses of a benzodiazepine. The risk of side effects, such as drowsiness and confused thinking, rises with increased doses of benzodiazepines.

When a person is physically or psychologically dependent on benzodiazepines, he or she can experience serious symptoms during withdrawal, including irritability, agitation, restlessness, insomnia, loss of appetite, tremor, muscle aches and, in some people, confusion or seizures. The danger of severe withdrawal symptoms can be diminished by using the smallest effective dose of a benzodiazepine for the shortest possible time and by slowly tapering the drug dose as it is discontinued.

Buspirone

The anti-anxiety drug buspirone (BuSpar) has fewer adverse effects than benzodiazepines, but it may be less effective, particularly for panic disorder. Common side effects of BuSpar are dizziness, headache, nervousness and nausea. However, BuSpar causes less drowsiness than other drugs, and abuse is unlikely because it does not lead to tolerance or dependence. In switching from benzodiazepines to BuSpar, a person may be able to minimize anxiety symptoms by starting immediately on BuSpar while tapering the dose of a benzodiazepine. For more on the drugs used to treat anxiety, see the chart on pages 60-61.

Herbal treatments

Kava kava, which is prepared from the crushed root of *Piper methysticum* (a shrublike pepper plant), is marketed as a natural remedy for anxiety and stress. However, the FDA has issued a warning that the supplement can damage the liver. In addition, long-term use of kava kava may result in allergic reactions, visual disturbances or difficulties maintaining balance. Kava kava should not be used if you are pregnant, breastfeeding or taking antidepressants.

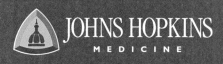

Valerian also is sold as a natural anti-anxiety remedy. Most research on the herb, which is prepared from the dried root of the plant *Valeriana officinalis*, has focused on people with insomnia. Less is known about its effectiveness in treating anxiety.

As with all herbal products, kava kava and valerian aren't regulated by the FDA, and there's no guarantee of their purity or effectiveness. Drug-herb interactions are also a concern. It is important to discuss all herbal remedies with your doctor before trying them.

Treatment of Specific Anxiety Disorders

Psychotherapy, medication and coping behaviors are used to treat all anxiety disorders. However, the disorders respond differently to the various treatment approaches.

Panic disorder

Treatment of panic disorder often involves both psychotherapy and medication. A therapist who specializes in treating panic disorder is best. According to a year-long study of 232 people with panic disorder treated at primary care clinics, sustained cognitive-behavioral therapy (gradual exposure to whatever brings on symptoms of anxiety) plus anti-anxiety medication is more effective than typical care (initial counseling and ongoing medication) for treating this type of anxiety.

Panic disorder may require more long-term drug therapy than other anxiety disorders (such as GAD). Tricyclic antidepressants and MAO inhibitors are sometimes used to treat panic disorder; both are 80 to 90 percent effective in blocking panic attacks but require six to 12 weeks to take effect. High doses of alprazolam (Xanax), a benzodiazepine, can be effective within a few days. While Xanax may cause fewer side effects than antidepressants, it is usually addictive (like all benzodiazepines).

In addition to benzodiazepines, the SSRIs fluoxetine (Prozac), paroxetine (Paxil) and sertraline (Zoloft) as well as the SNRI venlafaxine (Effexor) are FDA approved for treating panic disorder. The tricyclics desipramine (Norpramin), imipramine (Tofranil) and nortriptyline (Aventyl, Pamelor) also may be used, although they do not have FDA approval for treating panic disorder. Beta-blockers, such as propranolol (Inderal) or atenolol (Tenormin), can halt the physical symptoms of panic attacks but do not prevent the fear or panic itself.

Regardless of the specific drug(s) used to treat panic disorder, about 30 to 60 percent of people with the disorder suffer a relapse of symptoms six to 12 months after they stop taking their medication.

ASK THE DOCTOR

Q. *What is "exposure therapy" for phobias?*

A. This type of treatment for phobias involving certain situations, objects or animals requires people to confront the triggers of their fear. For example, someone with a phobia involving heights might climb to the top of a high building and look out the window. Someone with an extreme fear of snakes would be asked to touch one.

In some cases, the patient is exposed purposefully to these situations. A therapist first talks to the patient about how the phobia may have started and continued. Then the therapist carefully and gently encourages the patient to approach the fear-causing factor and remain there until the fear subsides partially or disappears. Once the intense anxiety has subsided, the therapist shows the patient how to continue to be exposed to the source of the problem to keep the phobia at bay.

Studies have found that after just 2 to 3½ hours of exposure, the majority of patients with phobias involving snakes, spiders, blood, claustrophobia, heights and flying had significant relief.

As another option, people with phobias may be able to use virtual reality technology to become accustomed to bothersome situations (like flying or heights) without real-life exposure.

Overcoming Social Phobia

How to face your fears and keep them from limiting your life

Sweating palms. Racing pulse. Ragged breathing. Nausea. We've all felt this way at one time or another in a stressful social situation, such as attending a funeral or speaking in front of a crowd. But you may feel this way all the time, even in the most ordinary encounters, like asking for assistance in a store or making small talk at a party. You may avoid interacting with others to the point where it seriously restricts your daily life.

If you're one of the 15 million American adults who experiences this type of fear, you should know that this is something more than just nerves—it's an anxiety disorder called social phobia.

Symptoms and situations

People with social phobia anticipate that interacting with others will be highly uncomfortable— that they will be embarrassed, judged, criticized or watched. This can manifest itself in physical symptoms like blushing, sweating, shaky voice or hands, muscle tension, confusion, nausea, diarrhea and heart palpitations.

Although any social situation can be stressful if you have social phobia, common triggers include attending parties, eating or drinking in public, making eye contact, ordering food in a restaurant, being introduced to strangers or using a public restroom. Social phobia can be limited to one specific situation (such as speaking in public) or can be

more general, to the point where people feel anxious around anyone other than close family.

People with social phobia know their fears are irrational and out of proportion, but they are unable to stop feeling that way. And they worry that other people will notice their anxiety, which makes it even worse. As the disorder can begin to take over their lives, it's not uncommon for co-occurring depression to result. Social phobia often leads to alcohol abuse, as many people turn to alcohol to ease their discomfort in social situations.

In a 2010 study, researchers examined data from the National Epidemiologic Survey on Alcohol and Related Conditions, for which more than 43,000 adults were interviewed during 2001 and 2002. People with social phobia were nearly three times more likely to be dependent on alcohol than the general population. Social phobia occurred before alcohol dependence in nearly 80 percent of cases, and it was associated with more severe cases of alcohol dependence and abuse.

Possible causes

People at risk for social phobias include those whose childhoods were characterized by shyness, solitude and a series of unhappy social experiences. Some evidence suggests that social phobia tends to run in families, but whether it's due to genetics or observing

other family members is unclear.

Researchers are investigating the role of the neurotransmitter serotonin, which helps regulate mood and emotions. It's possible that, similar to those with depression, people with social phobia may be sensitive to a serotonin imbalance.

There's also interest in the potential involvement in social phobia of the brain region known as the amygdala, which alerts the brain that a threat is present and evokes a frightened or anxious response in the body. For example, a 2010 study used magnetic resonance imaging to observe brain activity in people with generalized social phobia as well as those without the disorder. When they were shown socially threatening faces, people with social phobia exhibited greater activity in the amygdala.

When to seek help

If social phobia is interfering with your life—if you're avoiding people, places or situations because of your anxiety—it's time to see your doctor. Prepare for your appointment by writing down details about your symptoms (when they occur, when they began), your personal history (especially any changes that took place before symptoms began) and your medical history (including all health conditions and medications). Your doctor will perform a physical exam to rule out other causes of your anxiety

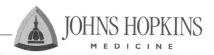

and may refer you to a mental health provider, who can design a treatment plan for you.

Social phobia is a chronic condition, although the symptoms do tend to come and go. But treatment can be very effective—80 percent of people with social phobia are able to overcome their fears when treated with medication, psychotherapy or both.

Medication. Medical therapy for social phobia depends on when your symptoms occur. If you have a phobia surrounding a specific situation—such as giving a speech or performance—your doctor may prescribe a beta-blocker such as propranolol (Inderal) to take just prior to the situation. Beta-blockers can lessen the physical expressions of anxiety (such as shaking hands or pounding heart) without impairing your physical ability to speak or move.

If your social phobia is more generalized, your doctor may prescribe an antidepressant, usually a selective serotonin reuptake inhibitor (SSRI) such as sertraline (Zoloft), paroxetine (Paxil) or fluoxetine (Prozac). These medications are well tested and have been proven effective for social phobia. SSRIs can take up to four to six weeks to begin relieving your anxiety. If needed, your doctor could prescribe an anti-anxiety medication such as alprazolam (Xanax), clonazepam (Klonopin), diazepam (Valium) or lorazepam (Ativan)—they promote calm and relaxation, and they work quickly. However, they can be sedating and are often habit-forming, so they're recommended for short-term use only.

Cognitive-behavioral therapy (CBT). A type of psychotherapy, CBT involves learning how to recognize and change negative thoughts and behaviors. It is helpful in up to 75 percent of people with social phobia. For many phobias, including social phobia, CBT may also include exposure therapy, which involves facing a series of increasingly anxiety-provoking situations. Steps may include spending time in a social situation or making small social blunders on purpose and observing people's reactions (which are usually not as severe as anticipated). CBT often lasts 12 weeks, and it can be done individually or in a group setting, which can be particularly helpful for social phobia.

In a 2011 study, researchers asked people with social phobia to give an impromptu speech while undergoing an electroencephalogram (EEG). The EEG revealed brain activity similar to that of a control group with high anxiety levels. After 12 weeks of CBT, a second set of EEGs (administered while giving another speech) showed that brain activity was now similar to a control group of people with low anxiety levels—suggesting that CBT may actually produce changes in the electrical activity of the brain.

Taking care of yourself
While social phobia can be best treated with medication and/or psychotherapy, there are steps you can take on your own to reduce your anxiety. First, try to identify the situations that make you most anxious: Is it dealing with people in a store? Sharing a meal with others? Making conversation? Then try to engage in these activities a little bit at a time. Ask someone for help in the grocery store, for example. Meet a friend for coffee or a snack, then gradually work up to a full dinner together. Initiate a conversation by asking someone about work or family.

You can also prepare for stressful situations in advance. Try reading up on a few interesting news items that you would feel comfortable discussing with people. Practice deep breathing to relax yourself. Remind yourself of all your positive traits—other people will notice them, too.

While you work on your mind, take care of your body as well. Regular exercise, adequate sleep and nutritious meals will help you deal with stress and anxiety. Try to avoid caffeine and other stimulants, which can increase anxious feelings. Avoid using alcohol as a social lubricant, and be sure to talk with your doctor or mental health provider if you have been using alcohol in this way. ■

Generalized anxiety disorder (GAD)

Despite its more chronic course, GAD responds better to treatment than does panic disorder. Psychotherapy helps many people, either by itself or in combination with medication. In addition, relaxation techniques, such as deep breathing exercises or meditation, may relieve symptoms of GAD.

The antidepressant medications Cymbalta, Lexapro, Paxil and Effexor are FDA approved for the treatment of GAD, but other serotonin and norepinephrine reuptake inhibitors, SSRIs, tricyclics, benzodiazepines and BuSpar also are commonly used to treat GAD.

Many people with GAD experience depression and self-medicate with alcohol, nicotine or other drugs, particularly benzodiazepines. As a result, someone with GAD who is being treated with a benzodiazepine should be given limited prescriptions of the drug (five to seven days). BuSpar, though sometimes less effective, may be a better option, as it does not cause dependence or withdrawal symptoms.

In terms of self-care, cutting back on caffeine may help ease the symptoms of GAD. One study found that the effects of caffeine, such as raising blood pressure, pulse rate and brain activity, were more pronounced in people with GAD. Moreover, people with GAD reported higher subjective levels of anxiety with greater caffeine intake.

Obsessive-compulsive disorder

As with panic disorder, OCD may improve with a combination of medication and cognitive-behavioral therapy. SSRIs, such as Celexa, Luvox, Lexapro, Paxil, Prozac and Zoloft, are now commonly used to treat this illness. The FDA has approved Luvox, Paxil, Prozac and Zoloft for the treatment of OCD (the first three are also approved for panic disorder). Improvements, which may take six to eight weeks of drug therapy, are more likely for compulsions than for obsessions. Higher doses of these medications (compared with those typically used to treat depression) may be necessary to treat OCD. Deep brain stimulation is available for severe cases of OCD for which medications and psychotherapy have not worked.

Post-traumatic stress disorder

Successful treatment requires a combination of psychotherapy—aimed at desensitizing the individual to the traumatic experience—and medication. A recent study in *Behavior Research and Therapy* found that eight to 12 sessions of cognitive-behavioral therapy (involving desensitization and progressive muscle relaxation) was better at reducing post-traumatic stress disorder symptoms than supportive therapy. Two SSRIs have been approved by the FDA for treating post-traumatic stress disorder: Zoloft and Paxil. The tricyclics Elavil and Norpramin are commonly used to treat the mood disturbances and anxiety that accompany the disorder.

Phobic disorders

When treatment is needed, cognitive and/or behavioral therapy may help desensitize the person to the thing or situation that causes the fear. Therapy involves gradually exposing the individual to the feared situation while teaching the person how to use various relaxation techniques to confront the fear.

Social phobia

Recent studies have shown that people with social phobia respond to the SSRIs Luvox and Paxil. Other SSRIs, such as Zoloft, and the extended-release serotonin and norepinephrine reuptake inhibitor Effexor XR may provide benefits as well. Tricyclics and benzodiazepines also may be used.

Many people who suffer from stage fright (such as classical musicians) use beta-blockers, like Inderal, for performance anxiety. Although the drugs may reduce the physical symptoms of performance anxiety associated with a particular event, they are not recommended for ongoing treatment. ■

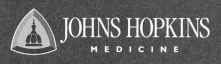

LATEST RESEARCH

Effexor XR for GAD Should Last at Least a Year

People with generalized anxiety disorder who are taking the drug venlafaxine XR (Effexor XR) should use the drug for at least a year, according to a new study.

Researchers from the University of Pennsylvania followed 268 people with generalized anxiety disorder (GAD) who began taking Effexor XR for six months. At the end of six months, the participants who improved were randomly assigned to keep receiving the drug for another six months or switch to placebo. When that second phase ended, those taking the placebo continued on it for another six months, and those who had been taking the drug either stayed on it or were switched to placebo, which became the third phase.

During the second phase, only 10 percent of participants who kept taking the drug for a year had a relapse of their GAD, compared with 54 percent of those who switched to placebo. In phase three, 32 percent of those who were taking the placebo for 12 months had a relapse, compared with 54 percent who had taken Effexor for only six months—suggesting that treatment with Effexor needs to be continued for one year to minimize the risk of a relapse.

These findings should help guide treatment with Effexor XR for patients with chronic anxiety.

ARCHIVES OF GENERAL PSYCHIATRY
Volume 67, page 1274
December 2010

agoraphobia—Fear of being in public places.

Alzheimer's disease—A progressive neurological disease marked by deficits in cognition, especially in memory.

antidepressant—A drug used to treat depression.

atypical depression—A type of depression in which a person does not experience sadness or some of the other symptoms normally associated with the disorder.

behavioral therapy—A form of psychotherapy that involves training in social skills, problem solving, scheduling of activities, and self-control. The emphasis is on day-to-day improvements in behavior.

benzodiazepines—A class of drugs used to relieve anxiety.

beta-blockers—A class of drugs used to treat angina, high blood pressure, irregular heart rhythms, and migraine. Chronic use of these drugs may cause depression; they are sometimes used in combination with antidepressants or to treat performance anxiety.

bipolar disorder—A mood disorder with episodes of depression and mania; also known as manic depression.

breakthrough depression—A depressive episode that occurs in someone with bipolar disorder or major depression who has been doing reasonably well with long-term treatment.

cognition—Mental abilities such as memory, attention, learning, awareness, and judgment.

cognitive therapy—A form of psychotherapy designed to reverse a person's belief that exaggerated weaknesses and inadequacies doom him or her to failure.

compulsion—Ritualistic, repetitive, and purposeful behavior that is performed according to certain rules or stereotypical patterns.

crisis intervention—See **interpersonal therapy**.

Cushing's disease—A medical condition caused by an overproduction of the steroid hormone cortisol by the adrenal gland.

deep brain stimulation (DBS)—A procedure in which an electrical stimulator (a pacemakerlike device) is implanted in the chest and programmed to send electrical impulses to a specific region of the brain. DBS is currently being tested for treating severe depression.

dementia—Deterioration of cognitive abilities resulting from a brain disorder or other disease.

depression—A mood disorder characterized by persistent low or sad mood, decreased or absent interest in almost all activities, loss of self-confidence, and a sense of worthlessness.

dopamine—A neurotransmitter; low levels are linked to depression and Parkinson's disease.

dopamine reuptake inhibitors—Antidepressant drugs that decrease the reabsorption of the neurotransmitter dopamine by the cell that released the dopamine.

double depression—Dysthymia with recurrent episodes of major depression.

dysthymia—A chronic disorder lasting two years or more, characterized by the presence of depressed mood for most of the day for more days than not. It may be intermittent, with periods of feeling normal, but relief lasts no more than two months. Symptoms are not severe enough to meet the criteria for major depression.

electroconvulsive therapy (ECT)—A series of sessions in which a controlled seizure is produced by attaching electrodes to the head and then sending brief electrical impulses through the skull into the brain. Used to treat depression and other psychiatric conditions when other treatments have failed or when immediate relief of symptoms is needed.

gamma-aminobutyric acid (GABA)—A neurotransmitter that suppresses the action of nerve cells. Decreased activity of GABA may contribute to anxiety disorders.

generalized anxiety disorder (GAD)—A condition characterized by persistent, excessive anxiety and worry.

glutamate—A neurotransmitter that stimulates nerve cells. High glutamate levels in the brain may contribute to depression.

group therapy—A form of psychotherapy in which people meet under the guidance of a therapist to share feelings, experiences, and solutions in a supportive environment.

Huntington's disease—A disease of the central nervous system characterized by jerky movements, personality changes, and dementia.

hypomania—Episodes of mild manic symptoms.

hypothalamus—A part of the brain located within the limbic system that regulates the pituitary gland and may be involved in hormonal imbalances sometimes associated with depression.

hypothyroidism—The condition of having an underactive thyroid gland. When untreated, it can trigger symptoms of a mood disorder.

interpersonal therapy—A form of psychotherapy that aims to help a person cope with immediate problems and difficult transitions (such as divorce). Also known as crisis intervention.

kava kava—An herb marketed as a remedy for anxiety; it is not approved by the FDA.

light therapy—A treatment for seasonal affective disorder (SAD) that involves exposure to sources of bright light.

limbic system—A group of structures deep in the brain that play a major role in processing memories and emotion. These structures include the hippocampus, amygdala, hypothalamus, and entorhinal cortex.

mania—A mood disorder characterized by elated or elevated mood, increased activity, overblown self-image, and exaggerated self-confidence.

manic depression—See **bipolar disorder**.

melatonin—A hormone that appears to play a role in the body's daily rhythms. In supplement form, it is marketed as a remedy for seasonal affective disorder. It is not approved by the FDA.

mixed state—A condition in bipolar disorder when simultaneous symptoms of mania and depression are manifest.

monoamine oxidase (MAO) inhibitors—Antidepressant drugs that increase brain levels of the neurotransmitters norepinephrine, serotonin, and dopamine by blocking the action of the enzyme monoamine oxidase, which normally inactivates these neurotransmitters.

neuroleptics—Antipsychotic drugs sometimes used to control the psychotic symptoms of bipolar disorder until other mood-stabilizing drugs begin to take effect.

neurons—Nerve cells in the brain.

neurotransmitters—Chemicals used for communication between neurons.

nonsteroidal anti-inflammatory drugs (NSAIDs)—A class of drugs (including ibuprofen and aspirin) that reduce pain and inflammation. NSAIDs can increase the risk of toxicity when taken with lithium.

norepinephrine—A neurotransmitter, low levels of which are linked to depression.

obsession—Recurring and persistent thoughts, ideas, images, or impulses, sometimes of an aggressive or violent nature, that invade a person's consciousness.

obsessive-compulsive disorder (OCD)—A condition characterized by recurrent, repetitive thoughts (obsessions), behaviors (compulsions), or a combination of both. A person with OCD recognizes that his or her obsessions and compulsions are unreasonable, intrusive, unnecessary, or foolish but cannot resist them.

omega-3 fatty acids—Polyunsaturated fatty acids that are found in certain foods, notably fish and flaxseed. Researchers are currently studying omega-3s as a potential treatment for depression and bipolar disorder.

panic disorder—A condition characterized by short-lived, sudden attacks of terror and fear of losing control; attacks begin without warning during non-threatening activities.

Parkinson's disease—A progressive neurological disease characterized by tremors, stooped posture, and slow movement.

phobic disorder—A condition characterized by persistent, irrational fears that significantly impair an individual's social or work performance.

pituitary gland—A small gland located at the base of the brain that releases hormones regulating growth and metabolism.

post-traumatic stress disorder (PTSD)—A form of chronic psychological stress that follows exposure to a traumatic event such as an earthquake, a violent crime (rape, child abuse, murder), torture, an accident, or warfare.

psychiatric nurse—A registered nurse, usually with a master's degree in psychiatric nursing, who specializes in treating mental disorders.

psychiatric social worker—A social worker with specialized training in counseling.

psychiatrist—A medical doctor trained in the diagnosis and treatment of mental disorders; psychiatrists are authorized to prescribe medications and hospitalize patients.

psychoanalytic therapy—A form of psychotherapy in which a person meets with an analyst three to five times a week in a stream-of-consciousness, free-association atmosphere that involves minimal feedback from the therapist.

psychodynamic therapy—A form of psychotherapy that focuses on the patient's previous experiences in an attempt to understand current conflicts or feelings about recent changes, such as retirement or grief.

psychologist—A person with a doctorate degree in psychology who is trained in counseling, psychotherapy, and psychological testing; psychologists are not authorized to prescribe medication or hospitalize patients.

psychotherapy—The treatment of an emotional, behavioral, personality, or psychiatric disorder by means of verbal and nonverbal communication, as opposed to the use of medication or physical interventions. Psychotherapy has many forms (see separate entries): interpersonal therapy; psychodynamic therapy; supportive therapy; behavioral therapy; cognitive therapy; psychoanalytic therapy; and group therapy.

rapid cycling—A condition that occurs in bipolar disorder and involves multiple episodes of depression and mania within a given year.

rapid transcranial magnetic stimulation (rTMS)—A procedure in which an electromagnetic coil is placed on the scalp and sends pulsed magnetic stimulation to the brain. rTMS is currently being tested for treating depression.

reuptake—The reabsorption of a neurotransmitter by the nerve cell that released it. Drugs that block reuptake allow the neurotransmitter in the synaptic cleft to continue stimulation of other nerve cells.

S-adenosylmethionine (SAM-e)—A supplement that is marketed as a treatment for depression; it is not approved by the FDA.

seasonal affective disorder (SAD)—Episodes of depression that occur during certain times of the year when there is less sunlight, usually beginning in November and lasting through the winter months.

selective serotonin reuptake inhibitors (SSRIs)—Antidepressant drugs that inhibit the reuptake of serotonin and thereby raise its concentration in the brain.

selective serotonin reuptake inhibitor (SSRI) withdrawal—Withdrawal symptoms experienced by about 25% of people who abruptly stop taking an SSRI. Most common symptoms are dizziness, nausea, lethargy, and headache.

serotonin—A neurotransmitter; low levels are linked to depression.

serotonin and norepinephrine reuptake inhibitors—Antidepressant drugs that inhibit the reuptake of serotonin and norepinephrine.

serotonin syndrome—A disorder that develops in some people who take a combination of drugs that raise the level of serotonin in the body. Symptoms include altered mental status and neuromuscular and nervous system problems.

social phobia—An undue fear of embarrassment in social situations. People with social phobia are so consumed by the fear of embarrassing themselves or being judged negatively that they avoid most social contact.

St. John's wort—An herbal remedy used for mild to moderate depression; it is not approved by the FDA.

supportive therapy—A form of therapy that teaches people about their illness, with the idea that a better understanding of the illness will enable them to set more realistic and tangible goals. The person's family members or close friends may be included in some counseling or education sessions.

synaptic cleft—The small gap between nerve cells; sometimes referred to as a synapse.

testosterone—The principal male sex hormone; it is currently being studied for its ability to treat depression in men.

tetracyclics—Antidepressant drugs with actions, effectiveness, and side effects similar to those of tricyclics.

tolerance—Decreased effectiveness of a given dose of a drug resulting from its continued use.

tricyclics—Antidepressant drugs that raise concentrations of the neurotransmitters norepinephrine and serotonin in the synaptic cleft by blocking their reuptake.

vagus nerve stimulator—A small, surgically implanted device that periodically stimulates the brain through the vagus nerve. It is used in the treatment of epilepsy and is being studied for treating depression.

valerian—An herb used to alleviate anxiety; it is not approved by the FDA.

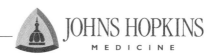

HEALTH INFORMATION ORGANIZATIONS AND SUPPORT GROUPS

American Association of Suicidology
5221 Wisconsin Ave., NW
Washington, DC 20015
☎ 800-273-8255 (crisis hotline)/
202-237-2280
www.suicidology.org
Publishes newsletters and journals on suicide prevention. Offers various services to suicide survivors.

American Psychiatric Association
APA Answer Center
1000 Wilson Blvd., Ste. 1825
Arlington, VA 22209
☎ 888-357-7924/703-907-7300
www.healthyminds.org
Medical society that provides patient information about mental illnesses, medication and psychiatric treatment.

American Psychological Association
750 First St. NE
Washington, DC 20002-4242
☎ 800-374-2721/202-336-5500
www.apa.org
Professional organization that publishes books, pamphlets and brochures on psychological issues.

Anxiety Disorders Association of America
8730 Georgia Ave.
Silver Spring, MD 20910
☎ 240-485-1001
www.adaa.org
Offers information on a variety of anxiety disorders and medications. Provides therapist referrals.

Depression and Bipolar Support Alliance
730 N. Franklin St., Ste. 501
Chicago, IL 60654-7225
☎ 800-826-3632
www.dbsalliance.org
Provides educational materials, support groups and a hotline staffed by people with depression or bipolar disease.

National Alliance on Mental Illness
3803 N. Fairfax Dr., Ste. 100
Arlington, VA 22203
☎ 800-950-6264/703-524-7600
www.nami.org
Advocacy organization dedicated to improving the lives of people with mental illness and their families.

National Institute of Mental Health
Science Writing, Press, and Dissemination Branch
6001 Executive Blvd.
Rm. 8184, MSC 9663
Bethesda, MD 20892-9663
☎ 866-615-6464/301-443-4513/
866-415-8051 (TTY toll-free)/
301-443-8431 (TTY)
www.nimh.nih.gov
Supports and conducts research on depression and other mental health disorders. Distributes information on various mental health disorders.

Mental Health America
2000 N. Beauregard St., 6th Fl.
Alexandria, VA 22311
☎ 800-969-6642/703-684-7722/
800-433-5959 (TTY)
www.nmha.org
Provides referrals to treatment services and support groups and offers literature on mental health topics.

INDEX

INDEX

NOTES

NOTES

NOTES

NOTES